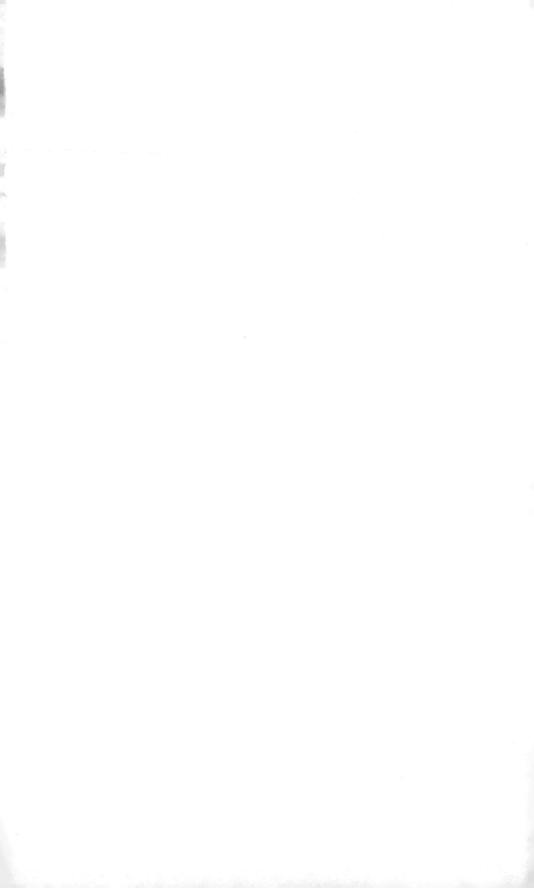

TUMOURS OF BONE

BY

WILFRED KARK

M.B., B.Ch., F.R.C.S.E., F.R.A.C.S. (Hon.)

Surgical Director, Workers' Rehabilitation Hospital, Johannesburg
Chairman, Examinations and Credentials Committee,
College of Physicians, Surgeons and Gynaecologists, of South Africa

BRISTOL: JOHN WRIGHT & SONS LTD.

1969

Distribution by Sole Agents:
United States of America: The Williams & Wilkins Company, Baltimore
Canada: The Macmillan Company of Canada Ltd., Toronto

SBN 7236 0247 6

PRINTED IN GREAT BRITAIN BY JOHN WRIGHT & SONS LTD.,
AT THE STONEBRIDGE PRESS, BRISTOL BS4 5NU

To Gilla, Charles, and David with deep affection and much admiration for the ways of the new generation

ACKNOWLEDGEMENT

THE substance of the first fourteen chapters of this book was published during the years 1967 and 1968 as a series of articles in *Medical Proceedings*. I have to thank the Editor of that journal not only for cession of the copyright to John Wright & Sons Ltd., but also for making available the original blocks.

Since publication in *Medical Proceedings*, the material has been revised and appreciable sections of seven chapters have been rewritten. Three new chapters, none of which featured in the original series, have been added to cater for certain regional peculiarities of bone and joint tumours.

CONTENTS

CHAPTER   PAGE

1. Classification, Incidence, and Diagnosis I

2. Benign Chondrogenic Tumours of Bone 10

3. Benign Osteogenic and Miscellaneous Group 26

4. Benign Fibrogenic Tumours of Bone 37

5. Chondrosarcoma 46

6. Osteogenic Sarcoma 53

7. Special Osteogenic Sarcomata 62

8. Fibrosarcoma of Bone 70

9. Giant-cell Tumour or Osteoclastoma 76

10. Ewing's Sarcoma 82

11. Bone Lesions in Malignant Neoplasms of Haemopoietic Tissues . 89

12. Malignant Vascular Tumours, Adamantinoma, Chordoma . . 99

13. Metastatic Carcinoma in Bone 106

14. Tumours of Synovium 112

15. Tumours of the Vertebral Column 118

16. Tumours of the Odontogenic Apparatus and Jaws 123

17. Tumours of the Hand 135

    Index 145

TUMOURS OF BONE

CHAPTER 1

CLASSIFICATION, INCIDENCE, AND DIAGNOSIS

CLASSIFICATION

PRIMARY tumours, arising from bone at one or other developmental stage, are to be distinguished from secondary bone tumours which originate by extension from tumours of neighbouring structures or by metastatic spread from more distant sites.

An aetiological classification of primary bone tumours is very desirable. It would obviously be useful in systematizing and clarifying pathology and in aiding clinical practice. However, it is not yet practicable because of the deficiencies in knowledge of causative factors. A regional division is practicable, but it is of slight value as bones and their tumours show relatively limited variations in different parts of the body. The conventional current grouping is based upon the particular bony tissue from which the tumour arises and, when such histogenesis is obscure, histological features are used in an attempt to complete the schematic arrangement.

In framing a classification, consideration of the behaviour of the tumour is superimposed upon the conception of its cellular origin. Thus, the natural course of tumours, whatever their precise origin, provides the important division into benign and malignant tumours.

The substance of such reflections on a schema for description of bone tumours is incorporated into the classification proposed by the Registry of Bone Sarcoma of the American College of Surgeons in 1928 and revised in 1939 (*Table I*, p. 2).

The Registry's histogenic formulation has provided a useful basis for comparative studies in different parts of the world. It has furnished a common language for correspondence and interchange of ideas, but it has several serious defects. Jaffe (1958) quotes the juxtaposition of chondroma and chondrosarcoma in the classification as exemplifying benign and malignant tumours in the 'chondroma series'. This implies a relationship between benign and malignant cartilage tumours which may not, in fact, exist. In regard to the 'benign chondroma', the classification fails to provide a clue to the marked clinical and radiological differences between benign solitary enchondroma and benign multiple enchondromata. Moreover, the more peripheral juxtacortical cartilaginous tumours, of both benign and malignant types, with their notable dissimilarities from the central enchondromata, are not catered for in the schema, which depends solely upon histogenic origins. Similar criticism is directed to 'osteogenic sarcoma' and 'exostosis'. Jaffe considers it preferable to avoid the Registry type of classification and, instead, to deal with a list of clinicopathological conditions as separate entities. His proposed list has the virtue of simplicity and correlation with clinical, radiological, and main histological features (*Table II*, p. 3).

I

Other authorities, recognizing the flaws in the Registry classification, have modified it so as to eliminate the more glaring inconsistencies and to incorporate later ideas. Phemister (1949) and Dahlin (1957) retain the core of histogenic origin in their classifications, but extend the listings of lesions to wider and more detailed proportions. Their elaborations appear to add complexity to the subject; whilst their lists are more complete, they detract from the value of a simple formula.

Table I.—CLASSIFICATION OF REGISTRY OF BONE SARCOMA (REVISED 1939)

	MALIGNANT	BENIGN
Osteogenic series .	Osteogenic sarcoma Medullary and subperiosteal Telangiectatic Sclerosing Periosteal Fibrosarcoma (*a*) Medullary (*b*) Periosteal Parosteal, capsular	Exostosis Osteoma
Chondroma series .	Chondrosarcoma Myxosarcoma	Chondroma
Giant-cell series . .	Malignant	Epiphysial giant-cell tumour
Angioma series . .	Angioendothelioma Diffuse endothelioma	Cavernous angioma Plexiform angioma
Myeloma series . .	Plasma cell Myelocytoma Erythroblastoma Lymphocytoma	—
Reticulum-cell lympho-sarcoma	—	—
Liposarcoma . .	—	—

Geschickter (1965a) bases his classification on the concept that tumour growth passes through the same stages as do normal processes of bone development and repair. According to him, nearly all neoplasms arise from an interruption of histogenesis; normal progress is blocked at some particular phase, which determines in large measure the type of tumour that results. This is constant for the stage of interruption and does not vary with the agent causing the block, whether this be congenital, hereditary, or acquired. The type of tumour additionally depends upon the duration of the interruption, as this influences the reaction of the tissues to the uncompleted normal development. Normal development consists of three major stages:—

Cartilaginous growth and calcification;
Resorption of calcified cartilage and giant-cell proliferation; and
Endosteal bone formation.

These phases are reflected in the main groupings of bone neoplasms.

Examples from another contribution by Geschickter (1965b) on mutations and congenital abnormalities in relation to bony neoplasms illustrate his concepts of definition and classification.

Table II.—BENIGN AND MALIGNANT PRIMARY BONE TUMOURS—
CLINICOPATHOLOGICAL ENTITIES (JAFFE, 1958)

MALIGNANT TUMOURS	QUASI-MALIGNANT TUMOURS	BENIGN TUMOURS

Osteogenic sarcoma
  Conventional
  Juxtacortical
Chondrosarcoma
  Central
  Peripheral
  Juxtacortical
Fibrosarcoma
  Well differentiated
  Poorly differentiated
	Giant-cell tumour	Osteoid-osteoma
		Benign osteoblastoma
		Fibrous dysplasia
		  Solitary
		  Polyostotic
		Chondroma
		  Solitary
		  Multiple
		  Juxtacortical
		Osteocartilaginous exostosis
		  Solitary
		  Multiple
		Desmoplastic fibroma
		Benign chondroblastoma
		Chondromyxoid fibroma
		Non-osteogenic fibroma

Malformations are gross anatomical deformities resulting from severe and drastic interference with normal growth during gestation or at birth. The conditions are not progressive and have no special tendency towards tumour formation.

Dysplasias arise from more subtle interruptions. The word connotes persistence of the phases of development reached at the time of the disturbance, and absence of the proper development of later stages. Many dysplasias exhibit a proclivity to neoplasia, as is exemplified by hereditary multiple exostoses and multiple enchondromata, congenital fibrous dysplasias, and acquired Paget's osteitis deformans, all of which have an excessive incidence of sarcomatous formation.

The concepts expounded by Geschickter are acceptable as an holistic, all-embracing explanation of the origin of tumours. The theoretical approach may indeed lead to a better understanding of oncogenic processes, but a classification distilled from it has no advantage over other systems in aiding clinical appreciation and management.

Up to the present, a universally satisfactory classification has not been evolved. Current knowledge does not permit of reasonable certainty in schematic arrangement according to genesis, histological pattern, or other pathological or clinical criteria. It would therefore seem preferable to adopt a simple formula and to maintain an open mind on the merits of other proposed systems. In the succeeding sections, bone tumours are considered in accordance with the following list (*Table III*, p. 4).

3

Table III.—Bone Tumours

Benign	Malignant
Chondrogenic:	Chondrosarcoma
Benign chondroblastoma	Osteogenic sarcoma
Chondroma—solitary, multiple, and periosteal	Special osteogenic sarcomata
Osteochondroma—solitary and multiple	Fibrosarcoma of bone
Osteogenic and Miscellaneous:	Giant-cell tumour
Osteoid osteoma	Ewing's sarcoma
Benign osteoblastoma	Reticulum-cell sarcoma
Solitary bone cyst	Multiple myeloma
Aneurysmal bone cyst	Malignant vascular tumours
Haemangioma	Adamantinoma of the tibia
Neural tumours	Chordoma
Fibrogenic:	Metastatic bone tumours
Fibrous dysplasia	
Chondromyxoid fibroma	
Fibrous cortical defect and non-ossifying fibroma	
Desmoplastic fibroma	

Special peculiarities of clinical presentation, unique types of pathological behaviour, and special problems of treatment are presented by tumours in certain sites. At the risk of a degree of repetition, particular sites—the vertebral column, the jaws and teeth, and the hand and fingers—have been added as separate chapters to gather together the special features of the tumours affecting them (Chapters 15, 16, and 17, pp. 118–144).

INCIDENCE

Based upon morbidity reports for 1949–51 in New York State, Goldberg, Levin, Gerhardt, Handy, and Cashman (1965) estimated the probability of developing cancer at all sites from birth onwards as 21·5 per cent in males and 25 per cent in females. To this total site probability, bone tumours contributed 0·110 per cent in males and 0·093 per cent in females. This means roughly that while 1 in 5 males and 1 in 4 females will probably develop cancer, 1·1 per 1000 males and 0·9 per 1000 females will develop bone cancer.

Harnett (1952) recorded somewhat higher incidences in a survey of 15,201 cases reported in London. In males, 0·93 per cent and in females, 0·81 per cent of the tumours were 'sarcomas of bone', that is about nine times the frequency estimated by Goldberg and his colleagues.

The National Cancer Institute (1958) gives the following relative incidence of primary malignant bone tumours (*Table IV*).

Table IV.—Relative Incidence of Primary Malignant Bone Tumours (National Cancer Institute)

Tumour	Percentage
Fibrosarcoma	7·2
Chondrosarcoma	8·3
Giant-cell sarcoma	5·0
Ewing's sarcoma	11·6
Osteosarcoma	38·1
Other sarcomata	15·5
Other malignant tumours	14·3

Differences in nomenclature account for divergences of figures in different series. *Table V*, of relative frequency of bone tumours (exclusive of metastases) at the New York Memorial Center, and modified from that given by Coley (1960), adds further light to the subject.

Table V.—RELATIVE INCIDENCE OF BONE TUMOURS
(NEW YORK MEMORIAL CENTER)

Primary Malignant Tumours Total: 1534 Cases		Benign Tumours Total: 790 Cases	
Tumour	*Percentage*	*Tumour*	*Percentage*
Osteosarcoma	39·3	Chondroma	16·7
Chondrosarcoma	17·9	Osteochondroma	33·4
Fibrosarcoma	5·8	Angioma	1·5
Ewing's sarcoma	14·5	Giant-cell tumour	13·6
Reticulum-cell sarcoma	3·2	Bone cyst	16·8
Myeloma	17·0	Chordoma	4·0
Giant-cell tumour	0·97	Aneurysmal bone cyst	3·8
Angiosarcoma	0·86	Fibrous dysplasia	7·46
Angioblastoma	0·46		

DIAGNOSIS

Clinical appraisal and laboratory investigations, roentgenography, and histopathology comprise the important approaches to the diagnosis of bone tumours. Although none of these tools of diagnosis is invariably reliable, the order given reflects, in ascending degree of importance, the relative contribution of each method to the final diagnosis. The clinical picture is only occasionally conclusive but is usually a pointer to one of a restricted set of possibilities. The radiological findings are more often determinative, but they are so beset by fallacies that they cannot be invested with unquestioning reliance. The histological picture is frequently diagnostically decisive but here, too, difficulties occur and misinterpretation may result. When all three approaches are correlated, the margin of error is considerably reduced and diagnostic accuracy reaches its highest level.

The following notes exemplify the leads to diagnosis given by the three methods of examination.

Clinical Features

AGE

Examples of the importance of age are seen in the following.

Osteogenic sarcoma has its peak incidence during late childhood and early adolescence. By contrast, chondrosarcoma is unusual at this period but commonly present during middle ages. A giant-cell tumour is rare under the age of 20 years.

DURATION AND PROGRESS

In terms of size and spread this may point to a slowly growing benign lesion or to a rapidly expanding and virulent malignancy. Measurement of the circumference of a limb aids appreciation of the progress of tumour growth. Occasionally it may demonstrate a sudden spurt in growth of a tumour which previously maintained a fairly constant size or very slow progression. The diagnosis of malignant transformation of a benign tumour is strongly suspect with such findings.

Symptoms and signs referable to organs other than the primary site may indicate the advent of metastases.

PAST HISTORY

This may include evidence of an earlier primary neoplasm and so raise the possibility of metastatic deposits in bone. In this connexion it is of value to inquire into and examine specifically those organs where carcinoma is known to have a proclivity to spread to bone, e.g., breast, kidney, prostate, lung, etc. The previous history may also contain references to non-neoplastic conditions, e.g., syphilis, osteomyelitis, typhoid fever, etc., which may have a bearing on the current condition.

THE FAMILY HISTORY

This may yield significant suggestions of hereditary dysplasias that are known to be tumorigenic. Hereditary multiple exostoses is an example of a condition with a disposition to sarcomatous change.

PAIN AND TENDERNESS

These raise suspicions of malignancy, and this is strengthened when there is rest-pain. Pain is often the herald symptom of bone malignancy. It may be mild and intermittent at the beginning and then become increasingly severe. Swelling and disability usually appear later than does pain. Benign bone tumours, with some exceptions, are seldom painful; when they are, it is usually the result of direct pressure on an adjacent structure, so that tenderness will be found in relation to this structure rather than to the tumour mass generally.

SITE OF TUMOUR

At times this is of help in directing attention to a probable diagnosis; or, in certain circumstances, it may lead to the elimination of some possibilities in a diagnostic field. It cannot be regarded as decisive as there are too many exceptions to the common situations.

The site of a bony tumour has two elements that bear on the diagnostic problem. The *location* of the tumour in relation to the major subdivisions of a long bone is one; the other is *the particular bone affected*. The following indicate the degree and range of importance.

Among benign tumours, osteoblastoma is most commonly situated in the vertebral column. Solitary enchondroma has a predilection for the metacarpals and the phalanges of the hand; in these bones, malignant transformation is rare. When the tumour affects long bones, malignancy is more likely to occur. Solitary osteochondroma, also named 'osteocartilaginous exostosis', usually arises near the epiphysis of a long bone, especially the lower metaphysis of the femur and the upper metaphysis of the tibia, and it grows away from the epiphysis.

A giant-cell tumour has so constant a situation in the great majority of cases that it is most unlikely to be the correct diagnosis if the lesion in a long bone does not involve the epiphysis.

Examples of predilection of site of sarcomata are shown in the following:—

6

Osteogenic Sarcoma: Femur in more than 50 per cent, and tibia and humerus in most of the remainder.

The metaphysis is most commonly affected.

Juxtacortical Sarcoma: This is so named on the basis of its situation.

Central Chondrosarcoma: This most commonly affects the metaphysis or diaphysis of the femur and, next, the upper metaphysis and epiphysis of the humerus.

Size, Shape, Definition, and Character of the Tumour

These may throw light on diagnosis. In general terms, the smaller the tumour, the more likely it is to be benign; and, since malignant growth is usually expanding, sarcomata become rounded or spindle-shaped. Appreciable definition of the margins of a tumour suggests benignancy; so too does absence of skin changes, viz., redness, local heat, thinning, and an increased vascular pattern. The presence of soft-tissue involvement, such as swelling, induration, and disturbed function, is a frequent accompaniment of malignant bone tumours.

Pulsation is an occasional finding. It denotes a very vascular tumour and one which involves, or has broken through, the cortex.

The consistence of bone tumours varies; it is not necessarily bony hard, but may be rubbery and surprisingly soft in rapidly growing sarcomata.

A General Examination

This may prove crucial in the diagnosis. Apart from the presence of constitutional effects of malignant tumours and its absence in benign neoplasms, the differentiation of non-neoplastic bone conditions, the presence of multiple bone lesions, and the discovery of a primary malignant tumour in soft tissues may be elucidated. The general examination should, of course, include standard and specially indicated laboratory procedures. The following examples emphasize the usefulness of this aspect of the examination.

A white-cell count may weigh in the differential diagnosis of inflammatory and neoplastic bone disease. A positive serological test for syphilis does not exclude a neoplasm, but it may clarify problems when added to the evidence brought to light by other forms of diagnostic survey. The serum calcium level is raised in the presence of bone destruction and decalcification, as in hyperparathyroidism and carcinomatous deposits in bone. If the alkaline phosphatase is within normal limits in the presence of bone tumour, then this is likely to be benign or of low-grade malignancy. A raised alkaline phosphatase suggests active bone destruction, as in metastatic carcinoma and highly malignant osteogenic sarcoma, or in Paget's osteitis deformans and in hyperparathyroidism. A high acid phosphatase directs attention to bone metastases from prostatic cancer.

Radiographic Evidence

Many of the features sought during the clinical examination will be subject to corroboration and elaboration by radiography. The following are among the more important radiological diagnostic elements:—

Accurate localization of the lesion is possible. The diagnostic utility of the precise location of a tumour has been indicated under the heading of Clinical Features.

7

The *extent* and *shape* of a tumour are important criteria. The direction and rate of progression of size are amenable to almost exact delineation. Extension into neighbouring structures, the manner of such extension, e.g., whether in regular form or along particular planes, and the gross shape of the lesion are often clearly depicted and serve as aids to diagnosis.

The *borders* of the lesion are revealed and their characters are weighty considerations in deciding their cause. Sharply demarcated lesions are usually benign, whereas infiltrating, unmarginated images of a tumour are suggestive of malignancy.

The fallibility of purely radiographic diagnosis is well illustrated in relation to these latter characters, as infiltration and the absence of clear margins may be found with inflammatory diseases, nutritional disturbances, and hormonal affections; and, on the other hand, clear-cut margins may be found in some malignant tumours, e.g., myeloma.

Shadow densities may be uniform or varied. Variations may arise from the matrix produced by some neoplasms, in some of which calcification and/or ossification may occur. Chondrosarcoma is an example of the production of a matrix in which flocculent, patchy calcifications occur. Osteogenic sarcoma commonly gives rise to an ossified matrix.

Variegated shadow densities are also due to bone destruction of different degrees, and the reaction of neighbouring bone to the lesion. Osteolytic activity varies in different tumours. The destruction by myeloma is not infrequently sharply defined; a giant-cell tumour may present a 'soap-bubble' picture; osteogenic sarcoma often destroys bone in a pattern indicating permeation. It is to be noted, however, that myeloma may present pictures with faint and vague outlines; and there are many records of giant-cell tumours which do not give a 'soap-bubble' sign, whereas some other conditions, like fibrous dysplasia and enchondroma, do quite often produce such shadows.

The reaction of the affected bone to the invading tumour may be proliferative. Periosteal and endosteal new bone formations occur. The grade of aggressiveness of the tumour is often suggested by the degree of organization of such new bone: the less malignant conditions tend to have a more or less encompassing reaction, whereas the more malignant conditions evoke a scattered, disconnected, and 'ineffectual' host-tissue reaction.

The characters of shadow patterns and densities are of substantial diagnostic import, but the reservation that there are no specific or pathognomonic radiological signs should be set against their importance. Radiography increases in significance when several coincident findings are interpreted in association with one another, and its validity is further improved when such a group of appearances is correlated with the clinical and pathological evidence.

Biopsy

The histopathological study of a representative segment of the lesion is very often crucial and decisive in the diagnosis. The examination may be done to confirm an opinion based upon clinical and radiographic assessment, or to add its quota of evidence when prior assessment has not passed beyond the stage of a debatable diagnosis. In the latter event it becomes mandatory. It is also essential before any patient is submitted to radical treatment, either surgical ablation, radio-therapy, or potentially toxic chemotherapy. There is an outside chance that a supposedly firm diagnosis derived from clinical and roentgenographic examination may be incorrect; radical therapy would be a tragic mistake, especially so when a biopsy might well have prevented it.

For the taking of a biopsy, both 'closed' and 'open' techniques are used; the former with a strong needle or special trocar and cannula, and particularly applicable to superficially situated bones; the latter by formal incisional approach and careful selection of the segment of tissue for biopsy removal. The element of careful selection of an exposed and visible portion of bone tumour and its immediate neighbouring tissues gives the open method a considerable advantage. The zone most likely to give definitive information can be better judged, and the vertical depth of the specimen, including portions of soft tissue, periosteum, cortex, and medulla, can be ensured to make the histological preparation more complete and more reliable. A surgical biopsy for immediate study of smears or sections is often done at an early stage of a planned operative procedure.

REFERENCES

COLEY, B. L. (1960), *Neoplasms of Bone*, 2nd ed. New York: Hoeber.
DAHLIN, D. C. (1957), *Bone Tumors: General Aspects and an Analysis of 2276 Cases*. Springfield, Ill.: Thomas.
GESCHICKTER, C. F. (1965a), 'Histogenesis of Bone Tumors', in *Tumors of Bone and Soft Tissue*. Chicago: Year Book Medical Publishers.
— — (1965b), 'Mutations and Congenital Abnormalities in Relation to Bone Neoplasms', in *Tumors of Bone and Soft Tissue*. Chicago: Year Book Medical Publishers.
GOLDBERG, I. D., LEVIN, M. L. GERHARDT, P. R., HANDY, V. H., and CASHMAN, R. E. (1965), 'The Probability of Developing Cancer', *J. natn. Cancer Inst.*, **17**, 155.
HARNETT, W. L. (1952), *Survey of Cancer in London*. London: British Empire Cancer Campaign.
JAFFE, H. L. (1958), *Tumors and Tumorous Conditions of the Bones and Joints*. Philadelphia: Lea & Febiger.
— — (1965), 'Histogenesis of Bone Tumors', in *Tumors of Bone and Soft Tissue*. Chicago: Year Book Medical Publishers.
NATIONAL CANCER INSTITUTE (1958), *The Extent of Cancer Illness in the United States*. U.S. Publ. Health Service Publ. No. 547.
PHEMISTER, D. (1949), 'Panel on Bone Tumors', *Proc. First Nat. Cancer Conf.*, p. 217. Washington: Am. Cancer Soc. and Nat. Cancer Inst. U.S. Public Health Service.

CHAPTER 2

BENIGN CHONDROGENIC TUMOURS OF BONE

THE following conditions are included in this chapter:—

Benign chondroblastoma.
Chondroma: solitary, multiple, and periosteal.
Osteochondroma: solitary and multiple.

BENIGN CHONDROBLASTOMA

Before 1942 this tumour was commonly linked to, and often regarded as a variant of, giant-cell tumours. Thereafter the proposition by Jaffe and Lichtenstein (1942) that it was a distinct and separate entity became widely accepted. The tumour probably arises from epiphysial cartilage and is characterized by its histopathological pattern.

INCIDENCE

It is uncommon.

AGE

It appears mainly during the second decade of life and is very uncommon below 10 or over 25 years of age.

SEX

Some series show a notably higher male incidence; in others, a more equal distribution is reported.

SITE

The main bones affected are the lower end of the femur, the upper end of the tibia, and the upper end of the humerus (*Fig.* 1). The tumour probably originates at or near the epiphysial line and spreads initially to involve the epiphysis and later the metaphysis as well. In the humerus and the upper end of the femur the usual sites of origin are the greater tuberosity and greater trochanter respectively.

PATHOGENESIS

This is unknown. One theory states that it is a development fault or mal-position of tissue.

CLINICAL PICTURE

Pain, tenderness, and swelling, all of which extend to the adjacent joint, are of moderate degree. Muscle wasting is usual and local heat is common. A limp may bring the patient for advice.

Radiographic Picture

The tumour has a round or ovoid shape, usually from 3 to 6 cm. in diameter. The site in the epiphysis, commonly extending into the metaphysis, is an important finding. The tumour is often central and causes expansion of the cortex which, in most cases, is asymmetrical. Periosteum overlying the affected cortex may exhibit proliferative reaction by the formation of new bone. The lesion is generally rarefied in an irregular pattern, with occasional trabeculation and, typically, mottled or patchy opaque areas due to calcification.

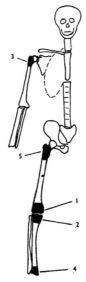

Fig. 1.—Sites of chondroblastoma in order of frequency in long bones. Sites 1 and 2 account for more than half the cases.

Morbid Anatomy

The tumour tissue is reddish grey and vascular in most areas; gritty and yellowish specks may be prominent. Areas of haemorrhage are usual, some of which exhibit organization or cystic replacement. The surface is often lobulated and the borders are clearly demarcated from surrounding bone.

Morbid Histology

The variegated histological findings probably reflect different phases of tumour activity. The chondroblast cells are polyhedral and fairly uniform in size; their nuclei are also uniform and regularly disposed in a central position. Scattered foci of calcification occur, not only in the ground substance between the cells, but also within the cells. The deposition of calcium brings about necrosis of the tumour cells, which then undergo connective-tissue replacement. Large vascular sinuses are found and haemorrhage is commonly associated. Adjacent to zones of necrosis with hyaline degenerative change and at areas of haemorrhage, clumps of giant cells appear. They constitute a cellular reaction to the changes

2

arising during the progress of the tumour, but they do not hide or disguise the fundamental chondroblast tumour-cell pattern.

DIFFERENTIAL DIAGNOSIS

Giant-cell Tumour
This is indicated in *Table VI*.

Chondrosarcoma
The main points are noted in *Table VII*, p. 13.

Enchondroma
See *Table IX*, p. 16.

Table VI.—DIFFERENTIAL DIAGNOSIS—BENIGN CHONDROBLASTOMA
AND GIANT-CELL TUMOUR

	CHONDROBLASTOMA	GIANT-CELL TUMOUR
Age . . .	10–24 years	20–40 years
Bones predisposed .	Lower femur, upper tibia, and upper humerus	Similar
Site within bone .	Epiphysis and metaphysis	Similar
Size . . .	3–6 cm.	Usually much larger
Radiography . .	Translucency more fuzzy with patchy densities	More clear
Histology Shape of cells .	Polyhedral	Ovoid and spindle stromal cells
Calcification .	Focal	Absent
Necrosis . .	Common	Absent
Giant cells . .	As 'foreign body' reaction; sparse small clumps	Numerous and widely distributed
General pattern .	Dominated by chondroblasts	Dominated by giant cells and stromal cells

TREATMENT AND PROGNOSIS

Complete extirpation by curetting is usually possible and, when achieved, is curative. Radiation therapy is not beneficial. Occasionally an apparently innocent chondroblastoma metastasizes to the lungs and behaves as a malignant tumour.

SOLITARY CENTRAL CHONDROMA

A not uncommon benign cartilaginous tumour occurs, as its name implies, as an enchondroma, i.e., central, and as a single lesion. It is also known as a 'solitary enchondroma'.

Table VII.—DIFFERENTIAL DIAGNOSIS—BENIGN CHONDROBLASTOMA
AND CHONDROSARCOMA

	CHONDROBLASTOMA	CHONDROSARCOMA
Site . . .	Central	May be central
Cells . .	Structure uniform	Pleomorphic
Nuclei . .	Uniform in size and position	Nuclei larger, irregular in shape and position, and hyperchromatic
Mitosis . .	Only occasional	High mitotic index
Cartilage . .	Not formed	Mature cartilage is formed

AGE

The main incidence is from 20 to 30 years.

SEX

The sexes are equally affected.

SITE

The tumour has a predilection for the short-long (i.e., short tubular) bones especially of the hands. It also affects other long bones and much less often the ribs, spine, and sternum. It usually begins in the metaphysis. *Fig.* 2 shows the main sites and their relative proportions.

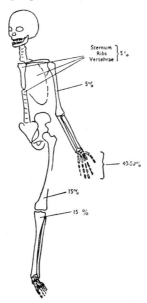

Sternum ⎫
Ribs ⎬ 5%
Vertebrae ⎭

5%

40-50%

15%

15 %

Fig. 2.—Solitary enchondroma. Common sites and approximate proportions.

13

Pathogenesis

This is unknown. As it is confined to bones formed in cartilage, it may come from a displaced cartilage rest.

Clinical Picture

A painless fusiform swelling of a phalanx or metacarpal/metatarsal is a common sign of its presence. It may be brought to light by slight trauma with pathological fracture, associated with pain and tenderness. The swelling is firm and smooth and may give the sign of 'egg-shell crackling'. Swelling also occurs in the lesions of the long bones and it may exist for years before causing any pain or disability.

Radiographic Picture

The lesion usually begins in the metaphysis and spreads to involve the diaphysis. It may extend into the epiphysis, but only after bony union has taken place. A spindle-shaped translucent tumour is usual in the tubular bones of the hands and feet. In addition to expansion, the cortex is often thinned and may be broken through by the tumour. Demarcation from unaffected bone is clear-cut. Small foci of calcification and ossification (from one to several mm. in diameter) disturb the uniformity of radiotranslucency and contribute a characteristic part of the picture. In the major long bones expansion is likely to be eccentric.

Morbid Anatomy

Lobulated islands of hyaline cartilage are prominent, partially or completely separated by connective and/or myxomatous tissue or simply by clefts. Areas of calcification and ossification are visible within the cartilage. The inner surface of cortex is eroded irregularly but smoothly; the outer surface is free of new bone formation except in areas of healing fractures.

Morbid Histology

Hyaline cartilage predominates. Cellularity varies but is seldom rich. The scattered cells are regular in form and content. Many are found in lacunae within wide areas of hyaline cartilage. Areas of calcification vary from aggregations of particles to substantial masses. Foci of ossification also vary in extent.

Malignant Degeneration

This very occasional event is more apt to arise in a long bone than in the bones of the hands and feet. It manifests by a fairly rapid spurt in growth of a tumour that has been either quiescent or slowly expanding for years. Histological evidence of the transformation may precede this clinical change by some months. Patchy increase of concentration of cells, irregularity of size and shape and nuclear content, and the advent of giant cells with large nuclei, all indicate malignant change. Cases have been recorded where malignant behaviour has occurred in the presence of apparently benign cytological appearance.

14

DIFFERENTIAL DIAGNOSIS

The most common solitary tumour of the tubular bones of the hands and feet is the enchondroma. Other conditions may cause confusion on the radiographic picture. *Table VIII* lists the main features of the more important lesions.

Table VIII.—DIFFERENTIAL DIAGNOSIS OF SOLITARY LESIONS IN SHORT-LONG BONES

	ENCHONDROMA	CYST	GIANT-CELL TUMOUR	OSTEO-CHONDROMA	FIBROUS DYSPLASIA
Incidence	Most common	Uncommon	Uncommon	Rarely solitary	Occasional. Seldom solitary
Site	Metaphysis (at least until union)	Inclusion cyst, mainly distal half of terminal phalanges	Epiphysis always affected	From metaphysis	Metaphysis
Calcification and ossification	Stippled foci are characteristic	Absent	Absent	Ossification by endochondral growth	Absent
Expansion of cortex	Usual; central and eccentric	Common	Particularly of articular surface and adjacent epiphysis	Projects as exostosis	Common
Demarcation	Defined	Defined	Defined	Defined	Absent
Rarefaction	Fuzzy light trabeculae	Trabeculation (in unicameral cyst)	Trabeculation may occur	Absent	Trabeculation common

Histological study is very often conclusive in differentiating the lesions. This is also true in regard to the diagnostic problems of solitary enchondroma in long bones. The main points are listed in *Table IX*, p. 16.

TREATMENT AND PROGNOSIS

Unsightly and symptomatic lesions call for surgical removal, usually by curetting. This is often accompanied by purposeful compression fracturing of the cortex; and, if this is insecure, by bone-grafts in single pieces or chips.

MULTIPLE ENCHONDROMATA

This is also commonly known as 'enchondromatosis' and 'Ollier's dyschondro-plasia'. The lesions consist essentially of cartilaginous tumours of different sizes disposed in several or many cartilaginous bones. It is uncertain whether the lesions are initially neoplastic. Many authorities favour cartilaginous dysplasia as the basic nature of the disease. The lesions may grow progressively and they show a proclivity to sarcomatous change.

Table IX.—Differential Diagnosis of a Solitary Lesion in Long Bones

	Enchondroma	Giant-cell Tumour	Chondroblastoma
Age	20–30 years	20–40 years	10–24 years
Site	Metaphysis at least until after union	Epiphysis spreading to metaphysis	Epiphysis and metaphysis
Size	Large	Large	Small
Radiography Translucency	Cloudy	Clear	Cloudy with patchy opacities
Calcification and ossification	Spotty	Rare	Irregular
Histology	Sparse cellularity and mature cartilage	Giant cells scattered in stroma-cell pattern	Chondroblast pattern. Giant cells in clumps

Multiple enchondromata are sometimes associated with haemangiomata; the name 'Maffucci's syndrome' is often applied to this association.

Incidence

The condition is uncommon. At the Memorial Center for Cancer and Allied Diseases, New York, solitary and multiple chondromata comprised 16·7 per cent of benign bone tumours (Coley, 1960).

Age

It is often first noted at about 2 years of age.

Sex

Males and females are equally affected.

Heredity

The evidence of hereditary disposition is slight and doubtful.

Sites

The chondromata arise only in bones formed in cartilage. Sometimes the bones on one side of the body are notably more involved than on the other. One or both metaphysial zones are commonly involved.

Histogenesis

Lesions arise from central cartilage and also from the deep layer of periosteum, whence they penetrate towards the centrum of the bone.

Pathogenesis

It is probably a disorder of cartilaginous development and growth. The cause of the disorder is not known.

Clinical Picture

Swelling and deformity are the most common initial manifestations and are often first observed in the fingers. Deformities of forearm and leg are frequent, arising from disturbance of proper growth of an affected bone. A limp may develop for the same reason. The tumorous growth may be very gross. Pathological fractures may occur but, apart from this, pain is unusual.

The most commonly associated soft-tissue lesions are haemangiomata. They may involve skin and/or deeper tissues and are not necessarily in the same regions as the affected bones.

Radiographic Picture

The tumours grow to distort and expand, or sometimes erode, the cortex especially in the metaphysis and diaphysis; occasionally at later stages the epiphysis is affected as well. The shadow is translucent, with irregular longitudinal linear markings of bony trabeculae. In some of the rarefied areas calcification produces spotty opacities.

Morbid Anatomy

Affected short-long bones are swollen in rounded or fusiform shape. Long bones are often bowed or even twisted in their long axis and shortened in length. Lobules and masses of cartilage of differing size, irregularly joined or separate, make up the bulk of the tumour. They may grow up to the cortical margin, to leave it relatively undistorted, or to bulge it into irregular tumefaction, or to penetrate it. Articular cartilage may exhibit warty excrescences.

Morbid Histology

The cartilage is much more cellular than in solitary enchondroma. Nuclei tend to be larger and more active.

Malignant Transformation

Jaffe (1958) estimates that more than 50 per cent of cases undergo chondrosarcomatous transformation in one or more sites of the lesion. Lichtenstein (1965) states that the risk of chondrosarcoma developing in enchondromatosis is great enough to call for constant alertness. Malignancy arises mainly during adult life, rather earlier than in primary chondrosarcoma but otherwise similar to it in cytology and behaviour.

Differential Diagnosis

The problem scarcely arises in view of the distinctive character of the multiple lesions. The relationship to, and the differentiation from, multiple osteocartilaginous exostoses are discussed under the latter heading.

TREATMENT AND PROGNOSIS

Individual deformities and disabilities may call for surgical and prosthetic assistance. Malignant areas may lend themselves to excision. Radiotherapy is of doubtful use in the benign state, but is helpful in malignancy.

PERIOSTEAL CHONDROMA

A chondroma, arising from cartilage adjacent to periosteum and replacing part of the bone cortex, occurs occasionally as a single tumour and more rarely in multiple form. The condition was proposed as a distinct entity by Lichtenstein and Hall in 1952. It is not so accepted by all authorities, some of whom regard it as a type of enchondroma.

INCIDENCE

It is a rare condition.

AGE

It is noted mostly during the third and fourth decades.

SEX

There is equal affection.

SITE

It affects short-long and long bones.

CLINICAL PICTURE

The usual presentation is as a painless swelling, often of many months' duration, and with growth so slow that it remains a small tumour. Tenderness is slight or absent.

RADIOGRAPHIC PICTURE

The usual diameter measures from 1 to 3 cm. Growth outside the bone profile produces a light shadow, commonly accompanied by cortical rarefaction which is clearly demarcated by sclerotic reaction. Denser shadows of calcification and/or ossification may occur within the tumour.

MORBID ANATOMY

The chondroma is encapsulated on its extra-osseous surface and is defined on its deep aspect. The lesion consists of lobules of mature cartilage, sometimes including calcified and/or ossified pieces.

MORBID HISTOLOGY

The cartilage cells are of uniform architecture and are more plentiful than in solitary enchondroma.

DIFFERENTIAL DIAGNOSIS

Two conditions, fibrous cortical defect and giant-cell tumour of a tendon-sheath, present certain radiographic similarities. The diagnostic features are listed in *Table X*, p. 19.

Table X.—DIFFERENTIAL DIAGNOSIS—PERIOSTEAL CHONDROMA,
FIBROUS CORTICAL DEFECT, AND GIANT-CELL TUMOUR OF TENDON-SHEATH

	PERIOSTEAL CHONDROMA	FIBROUS CORTICAL DEFECT	GIANT-CELL TUMOUR OF TENDON-SHEATH
Incidence .	Rare	Common	Rare
Age . . .	Adult	Childhood	Adult
Site . . .	Short and long tubular bones	Metaphysial cortex, especially lower femur	Mainly hands and feet
Radiography .	Sclerotic margin	Sclerotic margin	Erodes adjacent cortex
Histology . .	Lobules of cartilage	Whorled connective tissue	Connective tissue including cells containing cholesterol and pigment

TREATMENT AND PROGNOSIS

Surgical removal is usually possible and effective.

SOLITARY OSTEOCHONDROMA OR OSTEOCARTILAGINOUS EXOSTOSIS

The tumour consists of a single outgrowth of bony tissue with a cartilage cap at its free end. Frequently it is attached to the juxta-epiphysial zone of a long bone.

INCIDENCE

It is one of the commonest primary tumours of bone. The records of the Memorial Center, New York (*Table V*, p. 5) show that all osteochondromata contribute 33·4 per cent of benign bone tumours.

AGE

It usually appears during the first decade of life.

SEX

It is equally distributed.

SITE

Only bones formed in cartilage are affected. The lower femoral and the upper tibial metaphysis are the most frequent sites. Other fairly common sites are the upper end of the humerus, the lower end of the radius, and the lower end of the tibia.

PATHOGENESIS

The lesion probably arises from a displaced segment of epiphysial cartilage.

CLINICAL PICTURE

A symptomless lump is the usual herald. Friction or rubbing of structures in contact with the exostosis may produce pain, and tendon movement may be limited.

RADIOGRAPHIC PICTURE

The exostosis may have a narrow pedicle and present as a stalk with its free end bulbous and pointing away from the epiphysis; or it may be sessile with a bulky or squat protuberance (*Fig.* 3). The base is continuous, by cortical and medullary components, with the parent shaft.

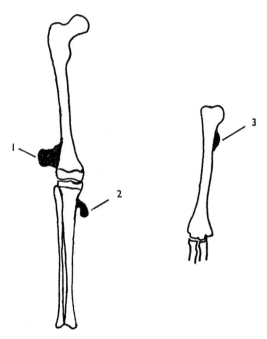

Fig. 3.—Solitary exostosis. Common sites of occurrence in order of frequency. The sessile type shown on the femur is reproduced from a radiograph of a girl of 19 years; the height of the exostosis exceeded the diameter of the related part of the femur. The pedunculated type shown on the tibia is commonly hook-like. The flat type is shown on the humerus.

MORBID ANATOMY

The exostosis is clearly defined and its situation, shape, and direction of growth are confirmed on naked-eye inspection. The expanded free end is capped by hyaline cartilage. The cap is more marked in younger subjects, tending to become progressively thinner and less extensive with increasing age, so that by the time of epiphysial union of the parent bone there are mere traces of the original cartilaginous plate. A bursa is not infrequent between the free end and the neighbouring soft tissues.

MORBID HISTOLOGY

The exostosis has a complete periosteal cover. A thin cortex is usual, the main bulk being composed of loose cancellous bone. These elements are continuous with those of the parent bone. Increase in size of the exostosis is by endochondral ossification, occurring *pari passu* with growth by ossification at the epiphysial plate.

MALIGNANT TRANSFORMATION

The development of a chondrosarcoma in a solitary osteochondromatous exostosis is very unusual. Jaffe (1958) estimates this at 1 per cent at most. When it does occur, it arises a decade or more after cessation of growth in size of the exostosis. Thus it is suspect when there is renewed enlargement after the age of 30.

SUBUNGUAL EXOSTOSIS

This condition is not a variant of an osteochondromatous exostosis. It arises most frequently from bone beneath the nail of the great toe and is probably occasioned by trauma.

DIFFERENTIAL DIAGNOSIS

This is considered under the next section on Multiple Exostoses.

TREATMENT AND PROGNOSIS

Pain, disability, and unsightly deformity are the usual indications for surgical removal, which is almost invariably curative. Sudden spurts in growth at older ages, indicative of possible malignant change, also call for surgery. In most cases of proven malignancy, surgical extirpation has been reported as successful.

MULTIPLE OSTEOCHONDROMATOSES OR OSTEOCARTILAGINOUS EXOSTOSES

This condition differs from solitary osteochondromatous exostosis, not only by its multiple lesions, but also in many other important respects, especially in that it is hereditary and it carries a high incidence of sarcomatous change.

INCIDENCE

It is not uncommon.

SEX

In many publications a preponderance of males in a ratio of 2 : 1 or 3 : 1 is described. This has been refuted by more recent studies (Solomon, 1964), which show an equal distribution.

HEREDITY

The findings of Stocks and Barrington (1925) that about two-thirds of cases were transmitted by an affected father and that, although unaffected fathers seldom transmitted the disease, unaffected mothers quite frequently did, have been brought into question by recent work (Solomon, 1964). Solomon's investigations included radiographic studies showing that females transmitting the disease were just as often affected as were male parents. Therefore, inheritance was in fact carried by a dominant gene and not, as might be suggested by the work of Stocks and Barrington, via a 'relative' dominant gene.

AGE

Most cases come to notice during childhood and adolescence.

SITES

The exostoses arise in bones formed in cartilage. The bones most commonly involved at an early stage are those about the knee-, ankle-, and shoulder-joints. The scapula, too, is often an early site.

PATHOGENESIS

Virchow, in 1891, advanced the theory that the lesions took origin from portions of cartilage separated off from epiphysial plates. Müller (1913) supported the concept of origin from cartilaginous nests derived from the deep layers of periosteum, which represented an abnormal function due to some general bodily upset. Keith (1920) regarded the condition as a failure of control, due to hormonal disturbance of the process of remodelling of bone, and accordingly designated it 'diaphysial aclasis'. Jaffe (1943) found signs in some specimens that there was failure by periosteum to produce the normal ring of bone which acts as part of the control of endochondral ossification. This evidence supported Keith's theory. Jaffe also found that periosteal function was further perverted in that it produced cartilage instead of bone, thus giving weight to Müller's periosteal theory. In fact, the two theories mutually reinforce each other.

The basic cause of the abnormal periosteal activity is regarded as being inherited.

CLINICAL PICTURE

The first clinical evidence is almost invariably the presence of multiple bony masses. The lumps, with few exceptions, remain free of pain, but grow gradually in size while others appear at fresh sites. When normal endochondral growth ceases, growth of the exostoses usually comes to an end.

Irregular bony outgrowths become conspicuous, especially in the metaphyses of the long bones. In them, too, shortening and bowing deformity are frequent. The narrow long bones, particularly the ulna and fibula, are often more markedly shortened than are their companion bones. In the forearm, this gives rise to a fairly characteristic deformity consisting of ulnar deviation of the hand, luxation of the head of the radius, and bowing of the forearm with its concavity on the medial side. Excessive shortening of the fibula causes tibial bowing with a convexity towards the outer side. Pelvic asymmetry is also frequent on account of different degrees of skeletal distortion on the two sides.

Increasing size of bony outgrowths may give rise to pain by pressure on neighbouring structures. Deformities of long bones may disturb the mechanics of related joints and cause arthritis, or they produce abnormalities of gait, thus adding symptoms to an initially asymptomatic condition.

RADIOGRAPHIC PICTURE

Most of the exostoses project from bones in the neighbourhood of epiphysial cartilage. Where the numbers and the rapidity of growth of exostoses are most marked, their general size and shape show the greatest irregularity. This is also applicable to the general architecture of the outgrowths: some preserve a regular bony pattern of spongy bone contained within cortex, as is found in solitary osteochondroma; others present whorled trabeculations or irregular densities arising from calcification. The metaphysis of a long bone is often expanded with its cortex irregularly thinned. The paired bones, especially so in the leg, may bear contiguous exostoses which become fused into a synostosis.

Radiography demonstrates that the elements constituting bony outgrowths run, without any break, into corresponding constituents of the parent bone.

MORBID ANATOMY

The variegated sizes, shapes, and gross structures of the exostoses have already been noted under the previous heading. In addition to the long bones, the scapulae, especially next to their vertebral borders, and the ribs are quite frequently involved. Less often, the iliac bones present outgrowths on both surfaces. Affection of the vertebrae is uncommon; when it does occur, it is the free ends of the spinous process that are involved. When there are widespread advanced lesions, the short-long bones of the extremities may be the seats of exostoses. The calcaneum is a not-infrequent site. Rarely, skull bones formed in cartilage present small, chondromatous, warty growths.

Cartilage caps cover much of the end surfaces of the exostoses. As in solitary exostoses, the caps are thicker and more extensive in younger subjects. Periosteum from the parent bone clothes the whole surface, including the cartilaginous portions. Cortical bone and the contained medullary tissues are continuous from parent to exostosis. The metaphysis is generally enlarged and modelling is distorted or entirely absent.

As in the solitary condition, bursae are commonly formed over the ends of multiple exostoses.

MORBID HISTOLOGY

The cartilage caps covering the exostoses are hyaline and from their deeper layers in young subjects the usual cellular pattern of endochondral bone formation is evident. Irregular patchy calcification of cartilage may be noted. In some cases, after the cessation of active bone formation, small discrete areas of cartilage remain as if trapped between bone trabeculae.

MALIGNANT TRANSFORMATION

The risk of the development of chondrosarcoma is high. Jaffe (1958) found it to be almost 20 per cent in one series of cases, and the supposition is that this figure would increase with the passage of time. Such secondary chondrosarcomata tend to present at a peak age of 40–45 years.

Increase in size of an osteochondroma after the normal age of completion of bony union across epiphysial plates is strongly suspect as pre- or actually malignant.

DIFFERENTIAL DIAGNOSIS

Multiple enchondromatosis presents diagnostic difficulties largely because of earlier theories that it was one variant of a cartilaginous developmental fault which also gave rise to osteocartilaginous exostoses; and, further, that the two chondrogenic lesions might coexist in the one case or in the one family.

Close investigation has negated this theory. They do not occur together. The two conditions are distinct and exhibit important individual characteristics. Some of these are listed in *Table XI*.

Table XI.—DISTINCTION BETWEEN ENCHONDROMATOSIS AND OSTEOCHONDROMATOSIS

	MULTIPLE ENCHONDROMA	MULTIPLE OSTEOCHONDROMA
Incidence . . .	Uncommon	Fairly common
Age of presentation .	Commonly 2–3 years	Peak is 10–24 years
Common site of presentation	Often first in fingers	Fingers—rare; most other bones formed in cartilage are commonly affected
Familial incidence .	Absent	Present
Heredity . . .	No evidence	Transferred as dominant factor
Site in bone . .	Within bone—central or eccentric, but no exostosis	Projecting exostoses are characteristic
Cartilage cap . .	Non-existent	Characteristic
Mixed lesions in one person or one family	Absent	Absent

TREATMENT AND PROGNOSIS

Cosmetic, symptomatic, and/or disabling considerations may call for surgical removal of benign lesions.

Secondary chondrosarcoma should be radically removed, if this is at all possible. If this is achieved, the prognosis is reasonable and not as serious as it is in primary chondrosarcomata.

Ionizing irradiation has not proved of value.

REFERENCES

COLEY, B. L. (1960), *Neoplasms of Bone*, 2nd ed. New York: Hoeber.
JAFFE, H. L. (1943), 'Hereditary Multiple Exostoses', *Archs Path.*, **36**, 335.
— — (1958), *Tumors and Tumorous Conditions of the Bones and Joints*. Philadelphia: Lea & Febiger.
— — and LICHTENSTEIN, L. (1942), 'Benign Chondroblastoma of Bone: A Reinterpretation of the So-called Calcifying or Chondromatous Giant Cell Tumor', *Am. J. Path.*, **18**, 969.

KEITH, Sir A. (1920), 'Studies on the Anatomical Changes which accompany Certain Growth-disorders of the Human Body', *J. Anat.*, **54**, 101.

LICHTENSTEIN, L. (1965), *Bone Tumors*, 3rd ed. St Louis: Mosby.

— — and HALL J. E. (1952), 'Periosteal Chondroma: A Distinctive Benign Cartilage Tumor', *J. Bone Jt Surg.*, **34A**, 691.

MÜLLER, E. (1913), 'Über hereditäre multiple cartilaginäre Exostosen und Ecchondrosen', *Beitr. path. Anat.*, **57**, 232.

SOLOMON, L. (1964), 'Hereditary Multiple Exostosis', *Am. J. hum. Genet.*, **16**, 351.

STOCKS, P., and BARRINGTON, A. (1925), *Hereditary Disorders of Bone Development.* Eugenics Lab. Memoirs 22. London: Cambridge Univ. Press.

VIRCHOW, R. (1891), 'Ueber multiple Exostosen, mit Vorlegung von Präpareten', *Berl. klin. Wschr.*, **28**, 1082.

CHAPTER 3

BENIGN OSTEOGENIC AND MISCELLANEOUS GROUP

THE following conditions are included in this chapter:—
    Osteoid-osteoma.
    Benign osteoblastoma.
    Solitary bone cyst.
    Aneurysmal bone cyst.
    Haemangioma.
    Neural bone tumours.

OSTEOID-OSTEOMA

The lesion consists of a small centrum of osseous tissue within a reactive bony sclerotic zone. Jaffe proposed it as a separate entity in 1935; in 1940 Jaffe and Lichtenstein recorded their further experiences and provided the description of the tumour that is generally accepted today.

INCIDENCE

By 1958 Jaffe reported a personal experience of 150 cases. The condition may be less uncommon than supposed. Symptomless, but otherwise typical cases have been revealed by radiography carried out for unrelated reasons.

AGE

Three-quarters of the cases appear during the age-group 10–25 years.

SEX

The ratio of affection is 2 : 1 (males : female).

SITE

The femur bears 25 per cent; the tibia 25 per cent; and almost every other bone has been reported (*Fig.* 4). It may arise in spongiosa or cortex.

PATHOGENESIS

This is unknown. Neither trauma nor inflammation plays a part.

CLINICAL PICTURE

Pain is the common herald, often occurring before the advent of radiographic manifestations. Localized, point tenderness is common. A small bony lump may develop at a later stage.

RADIOGRAPHIC PICTURE

The rounded centrum, usually relatively semi-opaque but sometimes dense, seldom exceeds 1 cm. in diameter. The surrounding bone is commonly thickened and sclerotic.

Morbid Anatomy

The lesion is obvious on naked-eye examination; its core is granular, reddish-brown, with occasional light mottling. In cortical lesions it may be hard and osseous.

Morbid Histology

The core consists of osteoid tissue and newly formed bone trabeculae in varying proportions, with a highly vascular stroma. It is clearly demarcated from its bed of surrounding bone. In lesions affecting the cortex, periosteal new bone formation around the centrum may be sufficient to form a swelling on the surface.

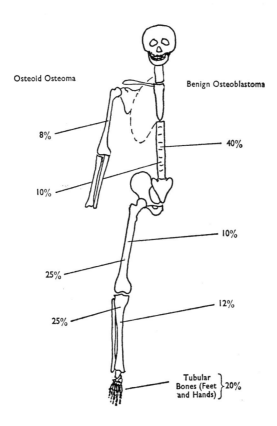

Fig. 4.—Osteoid-osteoma (right) and benign osteoblastoma (left). Approximate incidence at sites of predilection.

Differential Diagnosis
Medullary Osteoma

The features are given in *Table XII*, p. 28.

Table XII.—DIFFERENTIAL DIAGNOSIS—OSTEOID-OSTEOMA AND MEDULLARY OSTEOMA

	OSTEOID-OSTEOMA	MEDULLARY OSTEOMA
Pain and tenderness .	Present	Absent
Radiography . .	Reactive sclerosis	Opaque nidus without sclerotic surround
Histology of nidus .	Osteoid and osseous tissue	Mature bone

Osteoblastoma
See *Table XV*, p. 30.

Osteomyelitis
See *Table XIII.*

Table XIII.—DIFFERENTIAL DIAGNOSIS—OSTEOID-OSTEOMA AND BONE ABSCESS

	OSTEOID-OSTEOMA	BONE ABSCESS
Pain and tenderness .	Localized	More diffuse and intermittent
Fever . . .	Absent	Often present
Local heat . .	Absent	May be present
Leucocytosis . .	Absent	Usual
Histology . .	No evidence of inflammation	'Nidus' is a sequestrum or abscess cavity. Pus and inflammatory changes

Fibrous Cortical Defect
See *Table XVII*, p. 44.

Osteogenic Sarcoma
The central nidus of an osteoid-osteoma, when examined alone, divorced from its bony surround, may present a microscopic picture resembling that of osteogenic sarcoma. The main features in the differentiation are outlined in *Table XIV*, p. 29.

TREATMENT AND PROGNOSIS
Surgical removal of the centrum and surrounding zone of bone is curative. If removal is incomplete, the condition persists and gives rise to recurrence of symptoms after a varying interval.

Irradiation is not beneficial.

Table XIV.—Differential Diagnosis—Osteoid-osteoma and Osteogenic Sarcoma

	Osteoid-osteoma	Osteogenic Sarcoma
Size and progress .	Remains small	Grows expansively
Local reaction .	Sclerotic surround	Osteogenesis irregular if it occurs
Histology Cell . . . New bone . .	Regularity of structure Osteoid and osseous tissue	Irregularity and pleomorphism Atypical new bone formation

Benign Osteoblastoma

This is an uncommon tumour of vascular, osteoid, and osseous tissue, exhibiting many osteoblasts and favouring vertebrae for its most common situation. It has also been named 'osteogenic fibroma' and, on account of some similarity to osteoid-osteoma, Dahlin and Johnson (1954) named it 'giant osteoid-osteoma'. The different names applied to the condition are tokens of its ill-defined status.

Incidence

It is more uncommon than osteoid-osteoma.

Age

Most cases appear between 10 and 25 years.

Sex

There is no distinctive distribution.

Site

The vertebral body and arch take first place, followed by the short-long bones of the hands and feet. Other bones are also involved (*Fig. 4*).

Pathogenesis

This is unknown.

Clinical Picture

Affection of a vertebra gives rise to local pain and, by cord pressure, sensory and motor disturbances related to the level of the lesion. Radiating pain often becomes the dominant symptom. In the hands and feet, dull pain is followed by swelling. Pathological fractures may occur.

Radiographic Picture

The tumour expands the bone and varies in size up to a diameter of 10 cm. Translucency results from rich vascularity; parts may be dense with calcification; reactive sclerosis has been reported in lesions in the short-long bones.

MORBID ANATOMY

The tumour substance is gritty, interspersed with larger areas of calcification, and set in a pink-brown vascular stroma. Cortical bone may be penetrated.

MORBID HISTOLOGY

The characteristic finding is the presence of clumps and other aggregations of osteoblasts. In the richly vascular matrix, osteoid and osseous tissue are formed in varying proportions and osteoclasts are found at sites of resorption and development of osseous tissue.

DIFFERENTIAL DIAGNOSIS
Osteoid-osteoma

The similarities of cytological appearance have led some authors to the idea that the two conditions are phases of but one neoplasm. However, there are differences suggesting that they are two distinct clinicopathological entities. The main points of distinction are given in *Table XV*.

Table XV.—DIFFERENTIAL DIAGNOSIS—OSTEOBLASTOMA AND OSTEOID-OSTEOMA

	OSTEOBLASTOMA	OSTEOID-OSTEOMA
Site	Mainly vertebrae, then tubular bones hands and feet	Mainly femur and tibia
Size	Enlarges up to 10 cm.	Seldom exceeds 1 cm.
Pain . . .	Back pain, often with neurological disturbances	Localized to small area
Pathological fracture .	May occur	Absent
Histology . . .	Osteoblasts produce basic pattern	Osteoblasts in lesser proportion

Osteogenic Sarcoma

In particular, the osteogenesis in an osteoblastoma may, radiologically and histologically, raise a confusing picture. The absence of atypical pleomorphic and immature cells with many mitoses is the chief guide to eliminating a diagnosis of osteogenic sarcoma.

TREATMENT AND PROGNOSIS

Surgical removal, usually practicable in total measure for the bones of the hands and feet, but often only possible incompletely in vertebral lesions, is the treatment of choice. Following incomplete removal, X-ray irradiation is helpful and may induce healing.

SOLITARY BONE CYST

The cause of this condition is unknown. It is probably not neoplastic but the result of some traumatic or developmental disturbance.

INCIDENCE

It is uncommon. At the Memorial Center, New York, the relative incidence is recorded as 16·8 per cent of all benign bone tumours (*Table V*, p. 5).

AGE

The age-group 3–14 years encompasses about 80 per cent of cases.

SEX

Males predominate in a ratio of about 2 : 1.

SITE

The long bones are mainly affected. More than 50 per cent are found in the upper half of the humerus (*Fig.* 5).

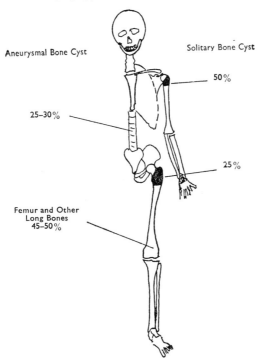

Fig. 5.—Solitary bone cyst (left) and aneurysmal bone cyst (right). Approximate incidence at sites of predilection.

PATHOGENESIS

This is not known. There are several theories, but with little or no supporting evidence for any of them. The supposition that it is a healing giant-cell tumour is negated by the absence of residual tumour tissue. Other theories linking the solitary bone cyst with diverse bone lesions, e.g., hyperparathyroidism and fibrous dysplasia, are subject to similar criticisms in that there is an absence of the full picture of these conditions in the solitary bone cyst. It is difficult to reconcile the common site of the cyst with the theory that it is an encapsulated residuum of a traumatic medullary haematoma.

CLINICAL PICTURE

Trauma with pathological fracture is the usual mechanism bringing the condition to notice.

RADIOGRAPHIC PICTURE

The cyst is found centrally placed, more often than not towards, and even abutting on, the epiphysial plate. The cortex is usually thinned and expanded on all surfaces in the region of the cyst, which extends down the shaft for a variable distance up to 3 in. or so. The radiotranslucent area is well defined: it may be loculated but there is no evidence of new bone formation.

MORBID ANATOMY

The cyst wall is a thin sheet of fibrous tissue. The cortex outside it is often so thin as to be translucent to the naked eye. The contents vary from clear to yellow and to blood-stained fluid, depending upon the occurrence and propinquity of recent trauma. The inner cortical surface presents ridges of different sizes which may account for some of the trabeculations seen on roentgen examination. Loculations may also be due to fibrous bands resulting from organizing thrombus from previous trauma.

MORBID HISTOLOGY

The thin lining is composed of a few layers of connective-tissue cells, with occasional patches of osteoid formation. The cortical wall has the appearance of periosteal new bone formation, a reaction to the resorption of the original cortex. Giant cells may be found near organizing blood and resorbing bone.

DIFFERENTIAL DIAGNOSIS
Aneurysmal Bone Cyst

The main points are noted in the following section under this title.

Giant-cell Tumour

Noted later, and summarized in *Table XVI*, p. 35.

Eosinophilic Granuloma

The radiological appearance may be confusing. However, an eosinophilic granuloma is usually small; it is often heralded by pain which then persists; and its histological characters, with eosinophils and histiocytes, all enable diagnostic separation from solitary bone cysts.

Monostotic Fibrous Dysplasia

Radiography may not provide means of differentiation, but the histological findings are decisive.

Treatment and Prognosis

Surgical curetting, bone chip grafting, and infracture of cortex, sometimes repeated, are curative in a great majority of cases. The recurrence rate after a first procedure is about 40 per cent; after a second procedure it is less than 5 per cent.

Ionizing radiation is of no value and it may be harmful at the young age at which the lesion occurs.

Aneurysmal Bone Cyst

The name was suggested to describe the ballooned-out appearance of the lesion and was first given an independent status by Jaffe and Lichtenstein in 1942. Some authorities, such as Edling (1965), regard it as one form of dysfibroplasia, in which group solitary bone cyst is included.

Incidence

It is more uncommon than is solitary bone cyst. The relative incidence at the Memorial Center, New York, is recorded as 3·8 per cent of benign bone tumours (*Table V*, p. 5).

Age

It is found mainly from 10 to 20 years.

Sex

It is equally distributed.

Site

The vertebral column and long bones are most commonly affected and account for 75 per cent of the cases. Of the long bones, the femur heads the list (*Fig. 5*), the common site within a long bone being in the metaphysial region.

Pathogenesis

Its common site at the metaphysial end of long bones and its main age incidence in adolescents point to the possibility of a disorder of bone formation. The fact that quite a number of cases are known to have disappeared after partial removal is evidence against it being neoplastic in character.

Clinical Picture

Swelling is usual and bulging into the pelvis has been described. Trauma may draw attention to the condition, but pain in the absence of injury also occurs. A vertebral lesion may cause symptoms referable to sensory and motor functions of a spinal nerve emerging from the canal near the cyst.

Radiographic Picture

The cyst causes what appears to be a blow-out of periosteum. The lesion is most commonly eccentrically placed in the metaphysis or diaphysis of a long bone, but this is not invariable. In slender bones, particularly in the fibula, as recorded by Tillman, Dahlin, Lipscomb, and Stewart (1968), the expansion of the bone is circumferential and roughly symmetrical.

33

The cortex is partly or wholly destroyed, so rendering the outer shell very thin and pencil-line on the plate. In the medullary portion of the bone an ill-defined zone of demarcation separates tumour from normal tissue. The cystic area is usually irregularly trabeculated.

The features described are essentially those found in long tubular bones, but in a vertebra the characters are obscure.

Morbid Anatomy

The cyst may grow to a large size, up to 3 in. (7·6 cm.) or more in long diameter. It is composed of multiple, irregular, communicating loculi, the walls of which may be soft or have thin, bony tissues giving them irregular segments of rigidity. The usual content of the loculi is blood in a fluid and fresh, venous form. When cut into or broken into at operative exploration, blood frequently wells up from the loculi suggesting that the cyst is made up of communicating vascular spaces, fed and drained by normal venous channels. This is not the invariable content of the cysts, as occasionally there may be blood-tinged or clear fluid within the loculi.

The outer shell is very thin and may consist of periosteum with only remnants of a bony shell. In the depth of the tumour there is no zone of sclerosis bordering its margins.

Morbid Histology

Periosteum, with or without a shell of bone, covers the blown-out tumefaction. The solid parts of the tumour, that is the tissues from the walls and partitions of the loculi, have many capillaries, fusiform connective-tissue cells, histiocytes containing haemosiderin, and, quite frequently, numerous giant cells of a 'foreign-body' type. The blood spaces are lined by endothelial cells which may be replaced in part by the cellular components of the walls between cysts. Parts of the walls of the loculi are composed of osseous tissue. It is important to stress the absence of muscle and elastic tissue such as is present in blood-vessels.

The cellular tissues as well as the cavernous spaces often extend completely through the cortex of the bone to lie immediately subperiosteally.

Differential Diagnosis

Solitary Bone Cyst and Giant-cell Tumour

The main features are given in *Table XVI*, p. 35.

Malignant Tumours of Vertebrae

The clinical and radiographic evidence often leave the issue in doubt, making microscopic examination essential for differential diagnosis.

Telangiectatic Osteogenic Sarcoma

Diagnosis may be very confusing on the basis of the radiological appearances and also the gross characters of the tumours. The finding of malignant cells and tissues is the final criterion for diagnosis.

Treatment and Prognosis

Surgical exposure and curettage, where feasible, is the treatment of choice. The residual cavity may require packing with bone chips. In inaccessible areas, partial curettage is usually done for diagnostic purposes but may lead to resolution.

Table XVI.—DIFFERENTIAL DIAGNOSIS—ANEURYSMAL BONE CYST,
SOLITARY BONE CYST, AND GIANT-CELL TUMOUR

	ANEURYSMAL BONE CYST	SOLITARY BONE CYST	GIANT-CELL TUMOUR
Age	10–20 years	3–14 years	20–40 years
Site	Metaphysis of long bone Mainly eccentric Femur particularly Vertebra common	Metaphysis of long bone Centrally placed Humerus particularly Vertebra uncommon	Epiphysis spreading to metaphysis Rare in vertebral column except sacrum
Radiography	Characteristic blow-out Cortex often absent Ill-defined separation from medulla	General symmetrical expansion Cortex thinned but present Defined deep limits	Large defined translucency
Content	Fluid blood—frequent, occasionally clear Appreciable soft tissue separating loculi	Clear yellow fluid, occasionally bloody Little or no tissue	Variegated solid, soft, friable, fleshy; later haemorrhages and necrosis may give cysts
Histology	Endothelial lining Rich capillaries and cellular elements in walls, extending to sub-periosteal level Osteoid tissue present Foreign-body-type giant cells	Connective-tissue lining Does not extend through cortex No osteoid Foreign-body-type giant cells	Plump round to oval stroma cells Scattered giant cells No osteoid or osseous tissue —

When recurrences follow incomplete removal, they usually become apparent within a few months. Further attempts at surgical extirpation often succeed.

Roentgen therapy is advocated and used by some authorities.

Sarcomatous degeneration has been reported. Tillman and others (1968) record the development of 3 sarcomata in 95 aneurysmal bone cysts. In the 3 cases, irradiation therapy had been used (such therapy was used either as an adjunct to surgical therapy or as the only therapy in 11 of the 95 cases). Chronic osteomyelitis and structural deformity are among the other complications of the condition.

HAEMANGIOMA OF BONE

VERTEBRAL

Symptomless haemangiomata are found in about 10 per cent of routine autopsies (Schmorl, 1927). Rarely, local and root pains, paralysis and vertebral collapse with paraplegia, occur. The roentgenogram is often diagnostic when the haemangioma is large enough to make an impression. A rarefied area with longitudinal striations of bone trabeculae is characteristic but not pathognomonic, as secondary myeloma and Hodgkin's disease may give a similar picture.

The haemangioma is almost always limited to the vertebral body. The larger lesions are more likely to be symptomatic. The vessels have a single-layered endothelial lining and are supported by oedematous fatty marrow tissue— cytological characters which are crucial in solving diagnostic problems.

Lesions occupying the main mass of a vertebral body have a special danger of potential collapse and spinal compression; this, and collapse itself, call for decompression by laminectomy. Apart from this indication for surgery, the treatment of choice is radiation therapy.

CALVARIAL

This is one of the sites for haemangioma. It presents as a painless swelling with a variable rate of growth. Radiographically, a sun-ray appearance is typical, closely resembling an osteogenic sarcoma.

From its original seat in the diploë, the haemangioma slowly rarifies and destroys the cortical plates. The outer periosteal layer covers the projecting mass, and on the inner surface, where growth is seldom pronounced, the dura remains intact. Bone trabeculae grow outwards, radiating from a centrum of irregular honeycombed bone and vessel pattern. Thin-walled vessels occupy the spaces between the bony spicules.

Surgical excision is curative and is possible in most cases. Radiation therapy stays the progress of the disease.

Other bony haemangiomata occur but are very rare.

NEURAL TUMOURS OF BONE

A Schwannoma is extremely rare within bone, and very few cases have been described. Neurofibromatosis is quite frequently a cause of bony lesions. Pressure on a bony surface gives rise to a smooth, hollowed-out defect; a neurofibroma of an intramedullary nerve produces a cyst-like rarefaction; scoliosis is featured in a number of contributions to the literature; curved deformities of the leg bones may arise congenitally; and other more uncommon lesions have a proved association with neurofibromatosis.

REFERENCES

DAHLIN, D. C., and JOHNSON, E. W., jun. (1954), 'Giant Osteoid-osteoma', *J. Bone Jt Surg.*, **36A**, 559.

EDLING, N. P. G. (1965), 'Is the Aneurysmal Bone Cyst a True Pathologic Entity?', *Cancer*, **18**, 1127.

JAFFE, H. L. (1935), 'Osteoid-osteoma: A Benign Osteoblastic Tumor composed of Osteoid and Atypical Bone', *Archs Surg., Chicago*, **31**, 709.

— — (1958), *Tumors and Tumorous Conditions of the Bones and Joints*. Philadelphia: Lea & Febiger.

— — and LICHTENSTEIN, L. (1940), 'Osteoid-osteoma: Further Experiences with this Benign Tumor of Bone', *J. Bone Jt Surg.*, **22A**, 645.

— — — — (1942), 'Solitary Unicameral Bone Cyst, with Emphasis on the Roentgen Picture, the Pathological Appearance and the Pathogenesis', *Archs Surg., Chicago*, **44**, 1004.

SCHMORL, G. (1927), 'Die pathologische Anatomie der Wirbelsäule', *Verh. dt. orthop. Ges.*, **21**, 3.

TILLMAN, B. P., DAHLIN, D. C., LIPSCOMB, P. R., and STEWART, J. R. (1968), 'Aneurysmal Bone Cyst: An Analysis of 95 Cases', *Proc. Staff Meet. Mayo Clin.*, **43**, 478.

CHAPTER 4

BENIGN FIBROGENIC TUMOURS OF BONE

THE following conditions are included in this chapter:—
Fibrous dysplasia—monostotic and polyostotic.
Chondromyxoid fibroma.
Fibrous cortical defect and non-ossifying fibroma.
Desmoplastic fibroma.

FIBROUS DYSPLASIA

The most notable effects of this condition are in bones, but often there are associated soft-tissue lesions in varying degrees and combinations. When skin involvement coexists, it manifests itself in areas of yellowish pigmentation. A small proportion of cases presents additional features: stunting of growth by early skeletal maturation, and precocious puberty (in girls)—a complex of features known as Albright's disease and indicative of a disturbed hormonal background.

Characteristic of the disease is the development of fibro-osseous tissue in one or more bones. The lesions are probably malformations rather than neoplasms; but the uncertain pathogenesis leaves the problem undecided.

In 1942 Lichtenstein and Jaffe separated the condition from a polyglot and muddled group, and named it 'fibrous dysplasia', a name which gives it a valid identity and avoids other confusing titles, e.g., focal or disseminated 'osteitis fibrosa' or 'fibrocystic disease', which encroach on descriptions of different bone diseases. When one bone is affected, these authors use the adjective 'monostotic'; 'polyostotic' applies to involvement of several bones. With extra-skeletal lesions, the eponym 'Albright's disease' is convenient.

INCIDENCE

The condition is not uncommon. The figure of 7·46 per cent of benign tumours of bone, given for the series at the New York Memorial Center (*Table V*, p. 5) appears to be lower than that suggested by Jaffe (1958). The monostotic is more common than the polyostotic form; and both skeletal forms are thirty to forty times as frequent as those combined with skin and other manifestations (Jaffe, 1958).

AGE

The lesions present particularly during childhood and adolescence.

SEX

Females preponderate in a proportion of 3 : 1.

SITES

Monostotic lesions are most frequent in the femur, tibia, rib, and jawbone. Schlumberger (1946) found rib involvement in 29 of 67 cases. Polyostotic forms are often confined to the bones of one lower limb. When the arm bones are involved, the skull bones often show stigmata. Occasionally ribs and vertebrae are the chosen sites. Severe cases tend to have a wide distribution, unilaterally or bilaterally.

PATHOGENESIS

In severe cases of Albright's disease, bony involvement is often remarkably unilateral, pointing to some developmental anomaly in its aetiology. Heredity has not been demonstrated as a factor.

Although the onset of precocious puberty in females, plus the occasional coincident hyperthyroidism, suggest a hormonal basis, this remains at present an unproven assumption.

CLINICAL PICTURE

This varies from a painless and unrecognized lesion to one giving pain, deformity and disability, as in the knee or hip region. Bones near the surface may exhibit a palpable and visible lump, as in a rib, the skull, or the jaw. Pathological fractures may bring the condition to light.

Polyostotic lesions present clinical features earlier than do monostotic ones. Widespread disease, especially when a fully developed Albright's syndrome eventuates, reveals itself in infancy, and advances to gross deformity, multiple fractures, and marked disability. Delay in starting or even inability to start to walk is common. Severe limping or a waddling gait may present at the earliest stage of walking.

Cutaneous lesions are flat and level with the surrounding skin and do not give rise to induration or thickening. They may be freckle-like or consist of larger, confluent patches of yellow to brown pigmented areas. Again, severe cases often present skin lesions at or soon after birth.

Epiphysial ossification and fusion may occur early, adding different degrees of dwarfism to that occasioned by spinal and lower limb deformity.

Severe cases may be associated with sexual precocity, which occurs more often and is more noticeable in females than in males.

RADIOGRAPHIC PICTURE

The general pattern shown radiographically varies with the relative amounts of fibrous and osseous components of the lesion. Osseous elements confer opacity, as is common in affections of the skull and facial bones; fibrous tissues are more translucent. 'Cystic' appearances arise from areas of cartilage set in the pathological fibro-osseous tissue, or from haemorrhage. The cortex is often expanded and thinned in an irregular and eccentric manner, and there is an absence of borders to the lesion. Erosion of cortex may leave ridges of more resistant bone, so producing a false picture of trabeculation.

MORBID ANATOMY

The affected portion of bone may be grossly swollen by 'tumour' growth which bulges and thins the cortex. Subperiosteal new bone follows the contour of the swelling. The outer surface is unbroken and smooth, but the medullary aspect of the cortex commonly presents irregular ridges. Radiographs depict these as trabecular lines which may falsely suggest the presence of bony loculi, whereas in fact the pathological tissue is usually fairly firm and solid, though not homogeneous.

Nodules of cartilage appear on the cut surface, especially at the metaphyses, as well as haemorrhagic and degenerative fluid cysts. Osseous ingredients within the 'tumour' tissue may be spotty and discrete or dense and sclerotic. The lack of defined margins to the abnormal tissue is evident.

With advance in age, osseous replacement continues until approximately the normal age of cessation of cartilaginous bone growth.

Morbid Histology

Different histological pictures are found in the several main components of the 'tumour'. Fibrous elements show whorled patterns of small spindle cells set in connective tissue. From parts of this tissue, varying amounts of bony trabeculae form. Some of the bony spicules undergo cystic degeneration, a change which is accompanied by the presence of many giant cells. Other areas show dense, closely set bone formation.

Malignant Transformation

Cases do occur, but they are uncommon (Coley and Stewart, 1945; Perkinson and Higinbotham, 1955). Osteogenic sarcoma and chondrosarcoma have been reported.

Differential Diagnosis

Several conditions are brought into consideration by the radiographic findings. When 'cystic' translucencies are prominent in monostotic fibrous dysplasia, a solitary bone cyst may be suggested; if the cartilaginous element preponderates in fibrous dysplasia, it may resemble the picture of a solitary chondroma; apparent trabeculation in fibrous dysplasia may simulate a number of bone-erosive conditions; multiple enchondromatoses, especially when the condition is conspicuously unilateral or confined to one limb, may raise problems of recognition; and widespread bone involvement in hyperparathyroidism may similarly cause difficulties in diagnosis. All these puzzling pictures are resolved by histological examination. Only fibrous dysplasia exhibits fibro-osseous tissue replacement, whereas the other conditions show their own cytological forms. Hyperparathyroidism is also differentiated by the associated blood chemistry; although cases of fibrous dysplasia may have a raised serum alkaline phosphatase, they do not show a raised calcium.

Differentiation of monostotic lesions from osteogenic sarcoma is noted in a later section. (Chapter 6, *Table XXI*, p. 58.)

Treatment and Prognosis

Pain and deformity are the main indications for surgery. Curettage and bone-grafting are suitable for long bones; partial resection for reduction of tumefaction is appropriate to jaw involvement; complete resection is applicable to localized lesions, as may occur in ribs; manipulation with immobilization may be required for pathological fractures; and supports and prostheses are used to aid various crippling deformities.

The more extensive and severe affections usually shorten life; mild forms, especially monostotic lesions, are compatible with normal longevity.

CHONDROMYXOID FIBROMA

This tumour is not chondrogenic in origin, but an intercellular development of chondroid character gives it the first part of its name. The 'fibroma' in the descriptive title is probably an accurate reflection of its connective-tissue origin. The myxoid features add the remaining element of the complex. Although the condition is rare, it has an importance in identification and separation from other bone tumours.

INCIDENCE

It is rare.

AGE

It presents mainly during the second and third decades.

SEX

There is an equal distribution.

SITE

It occurs mainly in the bones of the lower limb, especially the tibia. In a long bone, the metaphysis is most often affected.

CLINICAL PICTURE

Pain may be absent; when present, it is mild. The rate of growth is very slow and slight or moderate swelling is usually reported as having been present for a long time.

RADIOGRAPHIC PICTURE

The rounded, translucent lesions, with varying degrees of trabeculation, may measure up to 8 cm. in diameter. The margins may be vague in part and take the form of a sclerotic rim at other segments; on the cortical side, where there is expansion and thinning, periosteal reaction in the shape of an incomplete shell of new bone is often demonstrable. In the metaphysis of the tibia or femur the tumour is eccentric, involving only part of the circumference; in the fibula or in the bones of the foot, the tumour occupies more of the bone and is more central.

MORBID ANATOMY

Periosteal tissue appears to confer a surface capsule, and the deeper portions are clearly defined. The cut surface exhibits firm, elastic, whitish zones of chondroid, and greyish areas of myxoid set in lobules.

MORBID HISTOLOGY

The variety of tissues and the marked range of cytological appearances (with many of the stigmata usually attached to malignant tumours) raise considerable histopathological problems. This provides one of the exceptional examples where the radiological and, more particularly, the clinical evidence, outweighs histological findings in framing a diagnosis.

In the fibrous tissue partitions separating lobules of myxoid, there are profuse numbers of different sizes and shapes of cells with hyperchromatic nuclei. Within myxoid areas, cells are more sparse and exhibit nuclear variations. In parts, myxoid is replaced by collagen, presenting a chondroid picture whose similarity to cartilage may be more strongly suggested by the presence of cells within lacunae.

DIFFERENTIAL DIAGNOSIS

The important problem is the differentiation from chondrosarcoma, which is so forcibly suggested by the cytological picture, but which is susceptible to solution by evaluating the clinical and the radiological evidence.

TREATMENT AND PROGNOSIS

Surgical curettage is effective. Occasional recurrences usually respond to a second procedure.

FIBROUS CORTICAL DEFECT AND NON-OSTEOGENIC FIBROMA

The non-osteogenic, or non-ossifying, fibroma of bone is an advanced stage in the development of the condition known as 'fibrous cortical defect'. Although the early state is very common, the later 'fibroma' is not an inevitable sequel; in fact, it is infrequent.

Fibrous Cortical Defect

INCIDENCE

According to Caffey (1955), a high proportion of children are affected. Jaffe (1958) estimates it as high as 30–40 per cent.

AGE

It is most common from 4 to 8 years; and is rare under 2 or over 14.

SEX

Males predominate in a proportion of 2 to 1.

SITE

Solitary lesions are much more common than multiple ones; they are most often situated in the lower metaphysis of the femur; next, in the upper metaphysis of the tibia, then at either end of the shaft of the fibula. Other bones are seldom involved (*Fig.* 6). As the descriptive title implies, the lesion affects the cortex.

HISTOGENESIS

Jaffe (1958) reports studies indicating the origin from fibrous tissue derived from periosteum.

Pathogenesis

Caffey (1955) analyses the various theories, and considers that some local abnormality of development of periosteum is a more plausible explanation than local trauma or disturbance of bone growth originating in the epiphysial plate.

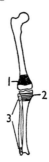

Fig. 6.—Solitary fibrous cortical defect. Sites of predilection in order of frequency. Few cases occur outside of these sites.

Clinical Picture

The condition is usually clinically silent, being revealed by radiological examination for some other purpose. Sometimes pain occurs. Occasional reports of pathological fracture have appeared.

Radiographic Picture

A profile view demonstrates the peripheral site of the lesion, growing into and eroding cortex. A different orientation of view may provide a false picture of a central cyst.

The translucent area is usually oval, with a longer vertical axis of 1–2 in. (2·5–5 cm.). A sclerotic rim bounds the deep portion, and its superficial surface is well demarcated. The sclerosis may extend in area, ultimately to obliterate the defect. Loculation is common in larger lesions.

Course

It is supposed that many fibrous cortical defects heal spontaneously; the fact that it is much less commonly found in adults than in children supports this assumption. Most lesions leave no trace; some are marked by an area of cortical sclerosis; a few persist, and, of these, still fewer proliferate to produce a non-ossifying fibroma. Jaffe (1958) reports having followed a few cases through the stages of transition.

Morbid Anatomy

Periosteal fibrous tissue in a restricted area is found growing into and replacing the underlying cortex. This is usually within half an inch or so of the epiphysial plate.

Morbid Histology

The fibrous tissue is continuous with periosteum and is arranged in whorled bundles. Sometimes collagen predominates; at other times the connective tissue is mature and it may be cellular with a scattering of giant cells. Lipid-filled cells may be a feature. The marginal sclerotic bone varies in density and thickness.

TREATMENT

The incidentally found, asymptomatic lesion does not require treatment. It should be submitted to routine periodic radiographic control. Painful lesions call for surgical curettage.

Non-osteogenic Fibroma

INCIDENCE

It is uncommon.

AGE

It is found mainly in the age-group 10–20 years.

SITE

Although the femur is the commonest site, it is not as predominantly the case as it is in the cortical defect. It lies in the metaphysis, usually eccentrically until late, when continued extension may bring it to the opposite side of the bone, or when narrow tubular bones are affected.

CLINICAL PICTURE

Pain, local tenderness, and swelling may arise spontaneously or follow trauma. The symptoms are usually of short duration (weeks or months) by contrast with the known long silent existence of the lesion.

RADIOGRAPHIC PICTURE

The site in the metaphysis is, more often than not, separated from the epiphysial line by a short distance. The translucent area extends from one side of the cortex to the centrum of the bony medulla in long bones of large diameter, but appears more centrally placed in a thin bone like the fibula. Bony trabeculae divide the rarefied zone into loculi of different densities and sizes. A soap-bubble or bunch-of-grapes appearance may be found in part of the affected area.

Demarcation is defined by a sclerotic rim in the depths, and by a thin bony shell on the outer surface over the area of eroded cortex.

EVOLUTION AND MORBID ANATOMY

Jaffe and Lichtenstein (1942) have clarified much of the pathological picture of the condition. In a minority of fibrous cortical defects the fibrous tissue continues to proliferate, reaching and excavating subcortical medullary tissue and constituting a non-ossifying fibroma.

The pathological tissue consists of nodes of firm fibrous tissue. Their colour is variegated, from grey to yellowish (when lipid-laden cells predominate) and to brownish (when haemosiderin deposition is marked). The nodes are irregularly separated by sclerotic bone or by strands of fibrous tissue.

The related cortex is often partially or completely destroyed but may also show increased density where, it is assumed, incomplete healing of the original cortical defect has occurred.

Morbid Histology

The whorled pattern of stromal spindle cells of the fibrous cortical defect is still in evidence. The cells are larger and more concentrated in some parts, especially where they contain haemosiderin. Giant cells are common but not plentiful; sometimes they are to be seen in clumps next to a haemorrhagic area. Lipid-laden foam cells are found in some tumours, but are not constant.

There is a reactive sclerosis of existing bony tissue around the whole tumour and in the shell defining some of the loculi, but there is no new bone formation within the connective tissues constituting the fibroma.

Differential Diagnosis

Periosteal Chondroma and Tendon-sheath Giant-cell Tumour

The main points in the differentiation of fibrous cortical defect from these conditions are given in *Table X* (p. 19).

Osteoid-osteoma and Cortical Bone Abscess

The main features are outlined in *Table XVII*.

Table XVII.—Differential Diagnosis—Fibrous Cortical Defect, Osteoid-osteoma, and Cortical Bone Abscess

	Fibrous Cortical Defect	Osteoid-osteoma	Bone Abscess
Age . .	4–8 years	10–25 years	Not significant
Site . .	Juxta-epiphysial	Varies	Metaphysis and diaphysis
Pain .	Absent	Marked and localized	Present, often intermittent
Size . .	Up to 3–4 cm.	Seldom more than 1 cm.	Small focus within dense cortex
Sclerosis .	Thin boundary	Marked	Marked
Histology .	Whorled connective tissue	Osteoid tissue marked	Inflammatory evidence clear

Giant-cell Tumour

Jaffe and Lichtenstein identified the non-osteogenic fibroma as a separate entity and thereby abstracted it from one of the supposed forms of giant-cell tumour. Nevertheless, the differentiation between the two conditions still presents occasional problems. The chief aids to diagnosis are listed in *Table XVIII*, p. 45.

Treatment and Prognosis

Curettage and bone chip grafts are often indicated and are successful. Recurrences are virtually non-existent.

Table XVIII.—Differential Diagnosis—Non-ossifying Fibroma
and Giant-cell Tumour

	Non-ossifying Fibroma	Giant-cell Tumour
Age . .	Usually under 20 years	Usually over 20 years
Site . .	Metaphysis	Epiphysis and metaphysis
Histology .	Whorled spindle stroma cells Intercellular substance often marked Small giant cells scattered, with few clumps	Stroma cells plump Intercellular substance minimal Large giant cells prominent and plentiful

Desmoplastic Fibroma

This designation was coined by Jaffe (1958) for a benign fibroblastic tumour, the cytological character of which resembles the desmoid tumour of the abdominal wall.

The condition is rare. It affects children and adults, and occurs in long and flat bones. It does not appear to involve the epiphysis. Swelling and mild pain usually call for radiographic examination, which shows a large, finely trabeculated, well-marginated, rarefied area. One segment of the cortex, or its whole circumference, may be thinned and expanded.

The firm, greyish, pathological tissue is composed of varying concentrations of small fibroblast cells with collagen fibres. The cells are of uniform size, shape, and internal structure, and mitotic activity is minimal.

Desmoplastic fibroma is at the benign end of a spectrum of fibroblastic tumours of bone. The spectrum then presents successive bands of fibrosarcomata, ranging from well-differentiated to very anaplastic types. Definitive diagnosis depends upon the cytological picture; this is not only so in differentiating it from fibrosarcomata, but also from other lesions, viz., chondromyxoid fibroma, non-ossifying fibroma, and fibrous dysplasia.

It is amenable to cure by curettage or resection.

REFERENCES

Caffey, J. (1955), 'On Fibrous Defects in Cortical Walls of Growing Tubular Bones', *Adv. pediat.*, **7**, 13.

Coley, B. L., and Stewart, F. W. (1945), 'Bone Sarcoma in Polyostotic Fibrous Dysplasia', *Ann. Surg.*, **121**, 872.

Jaffe, H. L. (1958), *Tumors and Tumorous Conditions of the Bones and Joints*. Philadelphia: Lea & Febiger.

— — and Lichtenstein, L. (1942), 'Non-osteogenic Fibroma of Bone', *Am. J. Path.*, **18**, 205.

Lichtenstein, L., and Jaffe, H. L. (1942), 'Fibrous Dysplasia of Bone: A Condition affecting One, Several or Many Bones, the Graver Cases of which may present Abnormal Pigmentation of the Skin, Premature Sexual Development, Hyperthyroidism or still other Extraskeletal Abnormalities', *Archs Path.*, **33**, 777.

Perkinson, N. G., and Higinbotham, N. L. (1955), 'Osteogenic Sarcoma arising in Polyostotic Fibrous Dysplasia', *Cancer*, **8**, 396.

Schlumberger, H. G. (1946), 'Fibrous Dysplasia of Single Bones (Monostotic Fibrous Dysplasia)', *Milit. Surg.*, **99**, 504.

CHAPTER 5

CHONDROSARCOMA

THE title is apposite to both histogenesis and dominant tumour cytology, for chondrosarcomata take origin from cartilage cells and then continue to produce neoplastic cartilaginous tissue. Primary chondrosarcomata probably arise *ab initio* from cells within the interior of the bone or more peripherally from or near periosteum. Secondary chondrosarcomata are superimposed upon previously benign tumours, particularly multiple osteochondromata and multiple enchondromata. Primary tumours are further subclassified into central and peripheral, in terms of their position in the bone involved.

Chondrosarcoma is less prevalent than is osteogenic sarcoma, the ratio being somewhat less than 1 : 2. Dahlin (1965) records that, at the Mayo Clinic, about 10 per cent of chondrosarcomata were secondary to osteochondromata and 1 per cent to enchondromatosis. Other authors place the ratios of secondary lesions at higher values. Most statistical analyses show that solitary chondrogenic benign bone tumours seldom become malignant, whereas the multiple conditions do so much more often.

PRIMARY CENTRAL CHONDROSARCOMA

INCIDENCE

Records, even in large series, vary. Representative examples of the incidence of all chondrosarcomata are those given by the National Cancer Institute (1958) as 8·3 per cent of primary malignant tumours of bone, and 17·9 per cent as recorded by Coley (1960) at the Memorial Hospital for Cancer and Allied Diseases, New York.

SEX

There is no notable difference in distribution.

AGE

Published records of age distribution vary considerably, probably because of the absence of an accepted uniform definition and classification. Jaffe (1958), taking primary and secondary central chondrosarcomata together, finds a range of 11–66 years with a median at 45. Coley (1960), considering primary chondrosarcomata of both central and peripheral situations together, reports the main range as from 10 to 25 years. He suggests that most of the tumours of this type that arise in later life are secondary transformations in original benign tumours.

SITE

The lower end of the shaft of the femur and the upper ends of the tibia and humerus are the commonest sites (*Fig.* 7). Other long and irregular bones may also be affected. The lesion may affect the mid-shaft or the epiphysis.

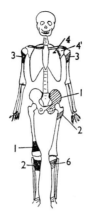

Fig. 7.—Common sites of primary (right) and secondary (left) chondrosarcoma. Sites 1, 2, and 3 of primary lesions account for about 70 per cent. The pelvis (site 1) is the seat of about 50 per cent of secondary tumours. The other numbered sites contribute about 40 per cent.

CLINICAL PICTURE

Pain is the common herald. It often increases in severity over a short period following a longer initial phase of relative mildness and intermittency. Swelling and disability become increasingly evident as the condition advances. Some traumatic episode may bring the condition to light.

RADIOGRAPHIC PICTURE

The tumour shadow is large, the bone diameter is often only slightly or moderately expanded, but it may (in rapidly growing lesions) extend beyond the line of the cortical shell into soft tissues. Characteristically, an irregular cloudy to light translucency is speckled in patches by varying numbers and sizes of radio-opaque spots. Disorderly loculation is not infrequent. Irregular destruction of cortex is usual; parts may be thinned, parts thickened, and yet others eroded. Periosteal new bone and the formation of Codman's triangles are quite common features.

MORBID ANATOMY

The tumour mass is composed mainly of irregular lobules of blue to grey-coloured cartilaginous tissue of varying consistency. Foci of calcification of irregular size and distribution show as white specks and give the cut surface a gritty feel. Extension along the medulla is usual, often involving at least a third of the length of the shaft. Extension into the epiphysis is quite frequent. Invasion of the cortex presents in different forms, all of which may occur in the one specimen. Erosive thinning, infiltrative thickening, periosteal raising with reactive new bone formation, and, in the more florid grades, frank penetration by tumour, all occur. The breakthrough may involve a joint, where spread (as in other soft tissues) is usually extensive.

Morbid Histology

Cartilage cells are the essential and dominant components. They are numerous and exhibit pleomorphism of cytoplasm and nucleus, marked nuclear hyperchromatism, many double nuclei, and occasional giant cartilage cells. Rapidly growing tumours often show a high grade of anaplasia, wherein spindle cells are prominent and give a picture of fibrosarcoma. Borderline cytological appearances may render the distinction between malignant and benign cartilaginous tumours uncertain. Often many areas require multiple sections before a confident diagnosis can be made.

Course and Spread

Tumour virulence varies. In children and adolescents, where anaplastic grades are more common, the progress of the tumour is rapid and tends to overwhelm the patient within 6 months or so after diagnosis. Differentiated grades may advance at a much slower speed, with limitation of local spread for many months and postponement of pulmonary metastases for some years.

The direction of local spread has been referred to under 'Morbid Anatomy'. Veins in the path of direct spread are invaded and tumour emboli are carried to the lungs, where metastases are common. Other forms of spread, lymphatic and systemic, are exceptional.

Differential Diagnosis

Benign Chondroblastoma

See Table VII, p. 13.

Enchondroma

Both solitary and multiple conditions raise diagnostic problems which are the more pressing as both forms, particularly multiple enchondromatosis, may undergo malignant transformation. The crucial question is the presence or absence of malignancy. Whether this has supervened on an innocent lesion or has been present *ab initio* is of secondary and minor importance. The solution depends mainly upon extensive histological examination. The main criteria of suspicion have been noted under the heading of Morbid Histology.

Chondromyxoid Fibroma

The lobules of chondroid and myxoid material may simulate, on gross and especially histological examination, a chondrosarcoma. The main differentiating factor is the innocent clinical course of chondromyxoid fibroma. In sites where chondrosarcomata are most common (femur, tibia, and humerus), the lesion involves the whole circumference of the cortex, as can be demonstrated radiologically; whereas chondromyxoid fibroma is eccentric, tending to affect only one part of the cortical surface.

Osteogenic Sarcoma

The points of differentiation are listed in *Table XXIII*, p. 59.

Treatment and Prognosis

Surgical ablation is not only the treatment of choice, it is also the only measure that has a chance of success. Local resections are almost invariably followed by recurrence, and radical amputations are therefore performed whenever possible. The tumours are insensitive to radiotherapy except in very strong dosage; thus this is reserved for palliation of inoperable lesions.

The prognosis usually varies directly with the grade of malignancy. Dedifferentiated and anaplastic lesions grow and spread rapidly, and there are but few recorded long-term survivals. Those that have recovered have followed early and radical amputations. In tumours of more mature cytological constitution, the prognosis is much better and survival has quite frequently followed a 'second' surgical ablation for recurrence after a 'first' more limited surgical attack.

Primary Peripheral Chondrosarcoma

The tumour begins in cartilage cells in or under the periosteum. Copeland and Geschickter (1965) regard this site of origin as the common one for primary chondrosarcoma generally; others consider it rare as the starting point for primary, but common for secondary lesions. According to Copeland and Geschickter, the tumour is initially mainly extra-osseous, invading cortex and medulla later. The picture thereafter is similar to that in primary central chondrosarcoma.

A number of features related to the aetiological, clinical, and radiographic aspects of this tumour are brought out in the next section on Diagnosis.

Differential Diagnosis

Multiple Osteochondromata

The distinction between primary peripheral chondrosarcoma and multiple osteochondromata is noted in *Table XIX*.

Table XIX.—Differential Diagnosis—Primary Peripheral Chondrosarcoma and Multiple Osteochondromata

	Primary Peripheral Chondrosarcoma	Multiple Osteochondromata
No. of lesions .	Single	Multiple
Pedicle . .	Absent	Often present
Radiography .	Generally translucent with opaque spots. First periosteal then cortical invasion visible. Later medulla destroyed. Periosteal new bone; often fine radiating lines	Cortical and medullary elements present. Parent bone cortex not invaded or eroded. No periosteal new bone formation
Histology .	Presence of malignant cartilage cells	Absence of sarcomatous cells

49

Secondary Chondrosarcoma

The differentiation between peripheral primary and secondary chondrosarcomata in exostoses is not an entirely academic subject. The prognosis of the primary sarcoma is much more serious than it is in secondary forms. Some of the main points are noted in *Table XX*.

Table XX.—Differential Diagnosis—Primary Peripheral Chondrosarcoma and Secondary Chondrosarcoma in Exostoses

	Primary Peripheral Chondrosarcoma	Secondary Chondrosarcoma
Age . .	10–25 years	35–55 years
Common sites .	About knee, and upper humerus	Pelvis provides 50 per cent; then mainly scapula, femur, and humerus
No. of lesions .	Single	One malignant lesion usual; but other sites show exostoses
Radiography .	General translucency with speckled opacities	Part of benign exostosis often still visible near malignant translucency
Progress . .	Usually rapid	Often relatively slow

CHONDROSARCOMA SECONDARY TO OSTEOCHONDROMA

This is included, by some authors, under the title 'peripheral chondrosarcoma'. Here, it is noted as a separate entity.

INCIDENCE

Malignant transformation of a solitary osteochondroma is exceptional, occurring in less than 1 per cent of cases. This is in distinct contrast to the incidence in multiple osteochondromata, where malignant change is not uncommon. Jaffe (1943) reported 11 per cent sarcomatous change in a series of 28 cases and suggested that, as the percentage would rise with increasing age of the cases, an incidence of 25 per cent was a reasonable estimate.

Dahlin (1965) reports that about 1 of 10 chondrosarcomata are secondary to osteochondromata, but other authors put the relative incidence higher. For example, Coley and Higinbotham (1954) report a much higher proportion of secondary lesions, amounting to about half the total number of chondrosarcomata.

HISTOGENESIS

The cell of origin is probably in the cartilage cap of the exostosis; or a subperiosteal cartilage cell lying away from the cap may be the starting point, as is sometimes suggested by the situation of the tumour.

AGE

It arises mainly in patients aged from 30 to 55 years.

SEX

There is a fairly equal distribution in the sexes.

SITE

The pelvic bones account for about half the cases. The upper portions of the femur and humerus, the scapula, tibia, and ribs provide most of the remaining cases (*Fig. 7*).

CLINICAL PICTURE

The change may be quite subtle, so that the patient (having been aware of multiple swellings for a considerable number of years) does not appreciate any special change in rate of growth at the site affected. Ultimately some rapid spurt in growth or the evolution of a gross enlargement brings the patient to medical care. Occasionally aggravation of pressure symptoms is marked; yet others are brought to light by some injury.

RADIOGRAPHIC PICTURE

Superimposed upon the picture presented by benign exostosis are the additional features of a cloudy translucent mass with opaque specks, and irregularly radiating striae from the centrum towards, and into, the soft tissues.

MORBID ANATOMY

The tumour is often large, from 6–10 in. (15–25 cm.) or more in one diameter. Its cut surface presents the typical lobules of cartilage, with patchy and spotty calcification, and there may be areas of haemorrhagic and cystic degeneration. Part, rather than all aspects, of the cortex is involved. Invasion of soft parts is generally late and slow.

MORBID HISTOLOGY

This is similar to that found in primary central chondrosarcoma, especially so at the less malignant end of the scale. The grade of malignancy tends to rise with successive recurrences following local surgery.

SPREAD

Direct spread tends to be slow and pulmonary metastases are often delayed for some years.

DIFFERENTIAL DIAGNOSIS

This has been discussed in the preceding section.

TREATMENT AND PROGNOSIS

In general these tumours have a better prognosis than have other chondrosarcomata. Thus more restricted radical resections are justifiable as a first measure. If there is recurrence, then amputation or wide ablative surgery is called for and it has many records of success.

CHONDROSARCOMA SECONDARY TO CHONDROMA

The incidence of this form of secondary chondrosarcoma is smaller than that associated with osteochondroma. Solitary enchondroma is seldom complicated by malignant transformation. When it does arise, it is less uncommon in a long bone than in the bones of the hands and feet. On the other hand, multiple enchondromatosis or Ollier's dyschondroplasia is frequently so affected, the incidence being variously estimated up to about 50 per cent. Not infrequently the sites of sarcomatous supervention are multiple.

The age-group, clinical features, cytological character, and prognosis are much the same as in other secondary chondrosarcomata.

Roentgenography is often of value in demonstrating fairly early sarcomatous change in a benign chondroma: a fuzzy shadow replaces part of the original benign picture and periosteum and cortex become involved.

REFERENCES

COLEY, B. L. (1960), *Neoplasms of Bone*, 2nd ed. New York: Hoeber.

— — and HIGINBOTHAM, N. L. (1954), 'Secondary Chondrosarcoma', *Ann. Surg.*, **139**, 547.

COPELAND, M., and GESCHICKTER, C. F. (1965), 'Cartilaginous Tumors of Bone', in *Tumors of Bone and Soft Tissue*. Chicago: Year Book Medical Publishers.

DAHLIN, D. C. (1965), 'Histogenesis and Classification of Bone Tumors', in *Ibid*. Chicago: Year Book Medical Publishers.

JAFFE, H. L. (1943), 'Hereditary Multiple Exostoses', *Archs Path.*, **36**, 335.

— — (1958), *Tumors and Tumorous Conditions of the Bones and Joints*. Philadelphia: Lea & Febiger.

NATIONAL CANCER INSTITUTE (1958), *The Extent of Cancer Illness in the United States*, p. 547. U.S. Publ. Health Service Publ.

CHAPTER 6

OSTEOGENIC SARCOMA

A DEGREE of confusion is inherent in the current use of two different definitions of this tumour. According to the American College of Surgeons Registry of Bone Sarcoma, the tumour derives from osteogenic cells and the name 'osteogenic sarcoma' is applicable, whether or not these osteogenic cells form osteoid or osseous tissue. A number of authorities disagree with this definition. In order to take account of several distinct forms of tumour, which may all arise from bone-forming cells and yet evolve into separate lines of behaviour, the connotation of an 'osteogenic sarcoma' is restricted to those sarcomata which do form neoplastic osteoid or osseous tissue. This may originate directly from the tumorous connective tissue or appear after an intervening cartilaginous phase.

This latter definition is used here. It has the advantage of permitting a fairly clear classification and separation of the entities osteogenic sarcoma, chondrosarcoma, and fibrosarcoma.

INCIDENCE

Platt (1952) estimates that bone sarcoma occurs in Great Britain in 1 of every 75,000 persons. Osteogenic sarcoma is the most common of the primary malignant tumours of bone, constituting about 40 per cent in many recorded series of large dimensions (*Tables IV* and *V*, pp. 4 and 5).

AGE

The peak age of incidence falls in the second decade of life; about 70 per cent occur in this period. Very few occur below 5 years or above 30 years. Cases that occur at ages older than 40 years are usually superimposed upon Paget's osteitis deformans or are consequent upon previous ingestion of a carcinogenic radioactive substance.

SEX

Males predominate in a ratio of about 2 : 1 (Dahlin and Coventry, 1967).

SITE

Whilst any bone may be affected, the sites of predilection are the lower end of the femur (accounting for between one-third and one-half of cases in different series), then the upper ends of the tibia and humerus (the former contributing almost 2 of every 10 cases, and the latter rather more than 1 in every 10 cases). About 10 per cent also occur in one or other of the bones forming the pelvic ring (*Fig. 8*).

In long bones, the tumour is commonly localized in the metaphysis. Spread, involving the epiphysis, is common. The lesion also presents in the mid-shaft.

PATHOGENESIS

Causative factors of the common form of osteogenic sarcoma are not known. In several unusual types of sarcoma, pathogenic agencies may be inferred. Whilst these are of great interest and may, in the future, prove important in providing a clue to the cause of the common variety, the findings and inferences in this small minority of special types cannot, as yet, be extrapolated to explain the circumstances affecting the majority. Against the background of this reservation, the following conditions having causative associations with osteogenic sarcoma are listed. They are noted more extensively in separate appropriate chapters.

Irradiated bone.

Paget's disease.

Fibrous dysplasia.

Giant-cell tumour.

Solitary enchondroma.

Multiple chondromata.

Multiple osteochondromata.

When malignant transformation does occur in the last three conditions listed, it is chondrosarcomatous rather than osteosarcomatous in character.

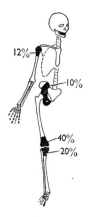

12%

10%

40%

20%

Fig. 8.—Relative incidence of osteogenic sarcoma at common sites of predilection.

CLINICAL PICTURE

The common herald is pain. Initially it may be mild, intermittent, and related to posture and exercise, but soon it grows in severity and becomes more persistent. In the area of pain there is a variable degree of tenderness, often extending from the end of the shaft and epiphysis to the related joint. Disability and limp may result.

Swelling is slight in the early stages and may only be discovered on comparative measurement of two limbs. However, increase in size is often rapid and this may bring the patient to medical care. A spindle-shaped swelling, affecting a third or half the length of a limb, indicates an advanced stage of tumour growth. The consistency of the swelling varies from case to case and in the same patient. Softness indicates haemorrhage and/or breakthrough into soft tissues. Hardness may vary in degree; with much tumour ossification, the mass will be 'bony' hard.

With advance in tumour extension an increase in local skin temperature and in the venous pattern may become noticeable. Haematogenous dissemination of sarcoma brings general constitutional changes: an ill and drawn facies, loss of weight, apathy, and lassitude often notify the impending fatal end.

Not infrequently the patient traces the onset of symptoms to some injury. This may present as a dramatic and distinct episode as in a pathological fracture, when radiographic examination surprisingly reveals the true pathology; or the association may be more vague and indefinite. Such a story raises the problem of trauma as a causative factor. Whilst there is as yet no final solution to the problem, the weight of evidence indicates that trauma acts by bringing the already existing tumour to notice and not as an inducing agent. In the rare instances where rigidly applied criteria permit a diagnosis of sarcoma after trauma, the probability of chance association is strong, a conclusion forcefully pointed by comparing the exceptionally rare positive examples with the enormous numbers of fractures and other bone injuries that are not followed by tumour formation.

LABORATORY FINDINGS

The alkaline phosphatase is frequently raised, more markedly as the tumour spreads locally and by metastasis. Both surgical and radiological ablative therapy tend to lower the serum level of alkaline phosphatase, unfortunately in most cases only temporarily. A later rise indicates reactivation; the higher the rise and, in fact, the higher the reading at any time from the onset of the disease, the worse the prognosis.

RADIOGRAPHIC PICTURE

Marked variations in appearance arise from different patterns of behaviour of the tumour. The variations are largely reflections of osteoblastic and osteolytic activity. Both forms of activity may occur in one case and there are many gradations in the range of behaviour of osteogenic sarcomata. In view of this, division of roentgenographic images into distinct classes is not, strictly speaking, justifiable, and only convenience of description excuses the following classification:—

1. *Osteoblastic, Sclerosing Type.*—Marked and extensive calcification and ossification are obvious radiographic features. The increased density affects an appreciable length (amounting to some inches) of medullary and cortical bone, often extending beyond the original cortex, which may still be apparent as a 'ghost shadow', to form an extracortical rounded, ovoid, or spindle shadow.

These radio-opaque zones often show recognizable forms of pathological and reactive new-bone production. As bone trabeculae are laid down at right-angles to the long axis of the bone, they give a picture of 'groomed whiskers' when short, and of 'sun rays' when longer. Such radiating spiculation is by no means constant or even very common with osteogenic sarcoma, and it may occur with other bone tumours.

In the area where the tumour shadow appears to bulge away from the cortex, especially so at the part distant from the metaphysis of a long bone, a periosteal cuff is often lifted away, forming a lip within which new bone is laid down so as to present a triangular shadow, often referred to as Codman's triangle.

Within the bone affected, there is an absence of a borderline to the process. There is, instead, evidence of an advancing, invading, and destructive tumour.

55

2. *Intermediate Osteoblastic Type.*—Radiotranslucent areas occupy a variable proportion of the total tumour shadow, indicating a mixed osteolytic and osteoblastic lesion. The translucency may affect both spongiosa and cortex, and it has no defined limits or regular pattern. Radio-opaque zones vary in intensity and extent; extracortical shadows may be woolly or heavy and dense, showing the patterns described under the 'sclerosing' type.

3. *Osteolytic Type.*—New-bone formation is absent or minimal and bone destruction of medullary and cortical zones produces the non-marginated, irregular rarefactions seen on roentgenographs. An important point in diagnosis is the absence of expansion or bulging of cortex.

Jaffe (1958) assesses the relative incidence in round figures of the three types as follows:—

Sclerosing type, 50 per cent;

Intermediate type, 25 per cent; and

Osteolytic type, 25 per cent.

The first two are usually amenable to diagnosis radiographically; the third group resembles the pictures produced by a number of other lesions and, therefore, raises major diagnostic difficulties.

PATHOLOGY AND MORBID ANATOMY

The same three classes of osteogenic sarcoma used to describe the range of radiographic evidence may be applied, with the same proviso of expediency, to the pathology of the tumour.

The tumour probably begins within medullary bone (a subperiosteal or juxtacortical variety is noted separately as it may represent a special form of osteogenic sarcoma), whence it spreads to involve surrounding cortex by the time of onset of clinical effects. Although the lesion is usually in the metaphysis, it may begin and spread from any part of the diaphysis. Extension from metaphysis to epiphysis is common. Advance from metaphysis along the diaphysis extends within the medulla, where the tumour tissue forms a plug with an apparent defined apex. In the cortex a limiting border cannot be appreciated.

Tumour-spread outside the line of the cortex often occurs before naked-eye evidence of complete breakthrough of the cortex. Initially this is limited to a subperiosteal zone, but later this layer, too, is transgressed. The ultimate tumour mass often assumes an oval or spindle shape. Part of the cortex, sometimes for lengths of several inches, is commonly completely destroyed and occupied by tumour tissue; none the less, traces or 'ghost remains' indicate the original cortical pattern.

The rubbery, grey-white areas of the lesion often contain yellowish patches and irregular lines of hard, gritty ossifying tissue. When this replaces most of the soft pathological tissue, the term 'sclerosing' is appropriate. In addition to neoplastic bone formation there may be other areas showing necrosis, haemorrhage, telangiectases, and cystic spaces. Mixed appearances fit the group classified as 'intermediate'; and when ossification is slight, the description 'osteolytic' is apposite. All varieties weaken the bone involved and pathological fractures are frequent.

SPREAD

Apart from direct spread to adjacent structures, blood-borne metastases to the lungs and occasionally to other parts of the skeleton occur. Fatal cases almost invariably have multiple metastatic foci in the lungs. Since most cases die within a year or so of diagnosis, spread to the lungs is not only common but very early. Bone secondaries appear mainly in the vertebrae, pelvis, and skull, suggesting involvement of the areas intimately concerned in the venous lakes and communications between the general systemic and the vertebral systems of veins. The anatomical studies of Batson (1942) and the mechanisms of interchange of venous blood are summarized in Chapter 15.

A few exceptional cases of lymph-node involvement have been recorded.

Morbid Histology

Osteolytic Type

The solid tumour tissues exhibit cells of different shapes and sizes. Spindle cells predominate, but there are also round shapes; some have barely discernible perinuclear cytoplasm, others are larger with much cytoplasm; and often there are areas showing marked anaplasia. Here, irregular mitotic activity is common. Giant cells appear by the formation of multiple nuclei which gather within a cell and enlarge it.

Osteolytic osteogenic sarcoma tends to spread rapidly, eroding and destroying spongiosa and cortex in its path. Not only is tumour osteogenesis meagre, but reactive bone formation by host tissues is noticeably slight or absent.

The tumour is highly vascular. Many vessels lined by tumour cells are formed; they often appear in more concentrated aggregations in some zones. The presence of large vascular cystic spaces led, in the past, to the description of 'malignant bone aneurysm'. Haemorrhages and necrotic areas are common.

Intermediate Type

Zones of the smaller cells may undergo cartilaginous differentiation, becoming plumper and rounded, and developing a lacunar surround. They usually remain in this state and ossification proceeds mainly or wholly by a membranous type of replacement, beginning by the formation of collagenous or connective-tissue strands set irregularly between groups and clumps of tumour cells. This forms osteoid tissue. As it increases in extent and thickness, stromal cells become trapped and, when calcification and then ossification replacement occur, the trapped cells diminish in size and appear as osteocytes. The whole process of ossification is irregular. Not only are the stromal cells between osteoid bundles pleomorphic and often anaplastic, but they are also grouped in varying numbers and in a disorderly manner. The connective-tissue strands and bundles are highly disorderly and irregular and the appearance of neoplastic bone is erratic and ragged.

In the intermediate type of osteogenic sarcoma, patchy new bone formation exists side by side with active areas of soft-tissue tumour and with 'cystic' zones of vascular channels, haemorrhages, and degenerative change.

At an early stage of spread, when the periosteum is slightly raised but still intact, reactive periosteal new bone may be laid down in the form of a few incomplete lamellae parallel to the original cortex. As periosteum is pushed out farther, new bone may be laid down at right-angles to the long axis of the affected bone, as if its disposition were directed by the stretched vascular channels between periosteum and cortex. These radiating spicules of irregular size and form are set in sarcomatous cellular tissue. Often new bone is formed without any pattern or dominant direction.

Sclerosing Type

Osteogenesis (neoplastic and reactive) is more dense and extensive. 'Soft' areas are restricted, and 'cystic' zones are sparse and small. By contrast with the rapidly advancing erosive destruction of an osteolytic tumour, the sclerosing osteogenic sarcoma is less vicious and eradication of host bone is relatively slow.

DIFFERENTIAL DIAGNOSIS

Osteoid-osteoma

See Table XIV, p. 29.

Monostotic Fibrous Dysplasia

When osseous replacement is marked in this lesion, difficulties arise in diagnosis. The main features of differentiation are summarized in Table XXI.

Table XXI.—DIFFERENTIAL DIAGNOSIS—OSTEOGENIC SARCOMA AND
MONOSTOTIC FIBROUS DYSPLASIA

	OSTEOGENIC SARCOMA	MONOSTOTIC FIBROUS DYSPLASIA
Age . .	10–20 years	Onset in childhood, but often presents in later years
Sex . .	2 males : 1 female	3 females : 1 male
Effect on cortex	No expansion, but destructive replacement and erosion through it	Expands and thins the cortex; but tumour confined by it
Histology .	Pleomorphism and grades of anaplasia	Whorled pattern of uniform spindle cells

Ewing's Sarcoma

Although neoplastic new bone is not formed, reactive new bone is laid down and roentgenograms may suggest an osteogenic sarcoma. The greater length of shaft involved, and the presence of lamellated subperiosteal new bone, when present in Ewing's tumour, help in diagnosis. However, it is the histological examination that provides differentiating evidence of greatest weight. This is referred to in greater detail in the section on Ewing's Sarcoma (Chapter 10).

Fibrosarcoma of Bone

Diagnostic difficulties arise mainly in relation to osteolytic osteogenic sarcoma. Table XXII (p. 59) lists the differentiating features.

Chondrosarcoma

The fact that chondromatous tissue is often found in osteogenic sarcoma may possibly lead to confusion with central chondrosarcoma. The main points of differentiation are given in Table XXIII, p. 59.

Table XXII.—Differential Diagnosis—Osteolytic Osteogenic Sarcoma and Fibrosarcoma of Bone

	Osteolytic Osteogenic Sarcoma	Fibrosarcoma
Age . .	10–20 years	Mainly in adults
Effect on cortex	Invasive destruction	Destroys but also thins and often bulges it slightly
Osteogenesis .	Some osteoid found; and traces of osseous change are not uncommon	Osteoid completely absent

Table XXIII.—Differential Diagnosis—Osteogenic Sarcoma and Central Chondrosarcoma

	Osteogenic Sarcoma	Central Chondrosarcoma
Age . .	10–20 years	10–50 years
Shadow .	Radio-opacities and translucencies may be mixed in one case but not in mottled or stippled pattern	Mottled radio-opaque foci in rarefied area
Cortex .	Destruction and replacement by tumour; no expansion	Bone expansion frequent in both primary and secondary forms; noticeable even with tumour breakthrough. The cortex is also often thickened
Pathological tissue	Cartilage may be present in limited areas, but the main components are varying proportions of greywhite soft material, osteoid and osseous tissues	The bulk is comprised of cartilaginous material; within which there may be foci of calcification or ossification
Histology .	Neoplastic osteoid and osseous tissues are characteristic	Complete absence of osteoid. Cartilage tumour cells are dominant

Metastatic Carcinoma

Both osteolytic and osteoblastic carcinomatous secondaries may give X-ray pictures simulating those of osteogenic sarcoma. The main points of differentiation are outlined in *Table XXIV*, p. 60.

Reticulum-cell Sarcoma

This rare tumour may resemble osteogenic sarcoma closely. The cytological composition is crucial in the differentiation.

Table XXIV.—DIFFERENTIAL DIAGNOSIS—OSTEOGENIC SARCOMA AND METASTATIC CARCINOMA

	OSTEOGENIC SARCOMA	METASTATIC CARCINOMA
Age . . .	10–20 years	Over 40 years
Other bone lesions .	Exceptional	Common
Main sites . .	Metaphysis	Mid-shaft
Histology . .	Diagnostic elements usually found	Cellular pattern usually points to primary origin

Inflammatory and Traumatic Conditions

Occasionally chronic osteomyelitis and myositis ossificans raise serious problems of diagnosis. A mis-diagnosis of osteogenic sarcoma may lead to radical treatment, a tragedy that is almost invariably preventable by histological investigation. Considerable difficulty may arise from the cytological picture of healing callus; correlation with radiographic study is of help.

PROGNOSIS

The somewhat arbitrary classification used to describe radiographical and pathological variants has some value in assessing prognosis. The sclerosing lesion has the best prognosis and the most favourable response to therapy; the osteolytic lesion is the worst. It seems, therefore, that prognosis varies directly with osteogenesis.

These general remarks on prognosis have to be read in the framework of an overriding qualification: osteogenic sarcoma has a sombre prognosis. The disease carries a high mortality. Statistical records of 5-year survival rate vary from 5 to 20 per cent, but differences of definition probably vitiate the more sanguine conclusions. Jaffe's assessment (1958) is at the lower end of this range, and personal experience is in accord with this figure.

TREATMENT

The results of treatment have been so gloomy that new tools and systems are constantly being sought. Surgical extirpation has become highly radical. Disarticulation of the hip-joint is practised for lesions of the lower end of the femur. Lesions with obvious extension to mid-shaft or more have been attacked by hind-quarter amputation. Similarly, tumours in the upper half of the humerus are commonly removed at a fore-quarter level. Occasional success may justify such far-reaching ablative procedures but, in general, the results have been depressing and disappointing.

In recent years attempts have been made to remove pulmonary metastases when they are localized to one focus, or to deposits in one lobe, or to one lung. The numbers are, as yet, too small to have significance, and more time must be allowed for appraisal of the value of such treatment.

Ionizing radiation was previously used when surgery was contra-indicated or when it had failed. It is now being tried as a more important weapon. New apparatus with higher voltage and greater power is under trial. Cade (1955) reports improved survival rates from the system of initial high concentration and dosage of radiation and, in those cases free of pulmonary metastases, later surgical ablation.

In 1964 Lea and McKenzie reported a trial of the following programme of management.

All new cases, except those with lung metastases, were accepted. High dosage of megavolt X-rays was given, followed by observation up to 3 months or more provided that clinical and radiographic improvement continued. Then, if the site of the tumour was suitable (e.g., in a limb) and if the lungs were free of metastases, surgical ablation was carried out. In cases with exceptionally good response to the radiotherapy, radical surgery was omitted from the programme. Of a total of 92 cases submitted to this trial, 20 survived for 5 years or more.

Barnes (1964), on the other hand, records disappointing results and suggests that primary amputation may be preferable for operable tumours.

Dahlin and Coventry (1967), taking into account only those cases first operated upon at the Mayo Clinic and only those without metastases when first seen, report just over 20 per cent 5-year survival rates and just over 17 per cent 10-year survivals. Studies of postoperative prognosis in relation to sex, tumour type, and grade did not point to any significant findings. However, location of the tumour had an important influence. Lesions distal to the upper end of the humerus carried a 25·4 per cent 5-year survival rate; the middle and distal segments of the femur had a lower rate of just below 19 per cent 5-year survivors; lesions below the knee- and elbow-joints had a 33·5 per cent 5-year survival rate. In the Mayo Clinic series the standard treatment for almost all cases in which it was practicable was radical amputation as early as possible.

REFERENCES

Barnes, R. (1964), *British Empire Cancer Campaign for Research. Annual Report*, p. 602.
Batson, O. V. (1942), 'The Role of the Vertebral Veins in Metastatic Processes', *Ann. intern. Med.*, **16**, 38.
Cade, S. (1955), 'Osteogenic Sarcoma', *J. R. Coll. Surg. Edinb.*, **1**, 79.
Dahlin, D. C., and Coventry, M. B. (1967), 'Osteogenic Sarcoma', *J. Bone Jt Surg.*, **49A**, 101.
Jaffe, H. L. (1958), *Tumors and Tumorous Conditions of the Bones and Joints*. Philadelphia: Lea & Febiger.
Lea, E. S., and McKenzie, D. H. (1964), 'Osteosarcoma', *Br. J. Surg.*, **51**, 252.
Platt, H. (1952), 'Symposium on Sarcoma of Bone, Royal Society of Medicine', *J. Bone Jt Surg.*, **34B**, 322.

CHAPTER 7

SPECIAL OSTEOGENIC SARCOMATA

JUXTACORTICAL OSTEOGENIC SARCOMA

JAFFE and Selin, in 1951, stressed the necessity for the delimitation of this lesion as a distinct clinicopathological entity. The reasons for differentiating it from conventional osteogenic sarcoma are outlined in *Table XXV*.

Whilst the tabulated features are those usually found, some exceptional juxtacortical osteogenic sarcomata behave in a much more hostile manner, invading the whole width of bone, breaking through rapidly and producing early pulmonary metastases. Geschickter and Copeland (1951) reported a new entity under the heading of 'parosteal osteoma'. They catered for the range of neoplastic behaviour by describing benign and malignant forms. This title has provoked objections because of its connotation of a benign tumour. Some authors, e.g., Dwinnell, Dahlin, and Ghormley (1954), use the designation 'parosteal osteogenic sarcoma'. Further confusion in nomenclature is added by others who agree with Willis (1960) in not accepting the lesion as a separate entity, but regard it as a variant of conventional osteogenic sarcoma.

Table XXV.—DISTINCTIONS BETWEEN JUXTACORTICAL AND
CONVENTIONAL OSTEOGENIC SARCOMA

	JUXTACORTICAL	CONVENTIONAL
Age	Mainly 10–50 years	Peak 10–20 years; few over 30 years
Site of origin	In or near periosteum	Central
Early growth	Oriented towards cortex	Involves whole width of bone
Rate of spread	Slow; even in late cases with medullary spread, further advance is slow	Rapid
Metastases	Often delayed for years	Usually early
Cytological appearance	Low-grade malignancy	High-grade malignancy
Alkaline phosphatase	Rarely altered	Often raised
Prognosis	Relatively good	Very poor

INCIDENCE

It is uncommon.

Age

The 2nd to the 5th decades of life are mainly affected.

Sex

The distribution is even.

Site

The lower femoral metaphysis, particularly its posterior region, is the most common site, accounting for about half the cases. This is followed by the other long bones, especially the humerus and the tibia (*Fig.* 9). It has also been reported in sites other than long bones.

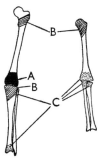

Fig. 9.—Juxtacortical osteogenic sarcoma: common sites. A. Solid black. Lower femur 50 per cent. B. Diagonal lines. Upper humerus, tibia, and femur 10–15 per cent each. C. Dots. Occasional sites in long bones.

Clinical Picture

Pain is often slight. Its persistence rather than its severity is likely to bring it to medical attention. In lower femoral lesions restricted flexion of the knee and swelling within the popliteal fossa are additional common features. Growth is slow, producing a defined bony-hard mass. The same features characterize recurrences after local excision. Such recurrences, in fact, often raise the index of suspicion, pointing to possible malignancy in a previously diagnosed 'benign osteoma'. Further recurrences may follow further limited surgery and they gradually assume more florid and aggressive characters.

Radiographic Picture

The tumour mass presents a dense shadow, projecting outside the line of the original cortex and occupying a large space in the soft-tissue areas; it may bulge the skin. The shadow is continuous with the original cortical density over a varying distance along one side of the bone shaft, and it may be mistaken for traumatic myositis ossificans. In neglected cases after prolonged growth, or after several local recurrences, and in the exceptional, more virulent variety, invasion of the medulla and involvement of the greater part of cortical circumference are demonstrable radiologically.

Morbid Anatomy

At a first surgical exposure the lesion appears well encapsulated, uniformly bony-hard, smooth or slightly lobulated on its surface, and firmly fixed to the related bone. Late cases, recurrences, and the exceptional high-grade malignant types, exhibit irregularities. These tumours may invade surrounding soft tissues as well as erode and destroy bone.

Section through the early lesion shows the heavily ossified tumour to be continuous with part of the cortex; sometimes only with periosteum and apparently separable from cortex. It is such cases particularly that tempt the surgeon to undertake limited local removal, with the almost certain sequel of recurrence. Section of the specimen also demonstrates fibrous areas (some of which are undergoing calcification), occasional cartilaginous foci, and the dominant bony tissue.

MORBID HISTOLOGY

A wide range of histological findings has been reported. Variation is not only apparent in different cases, but also in a single tumour. Soft-tissue zones may exhibit fibrous tissues in different arrangements and patterns. Cellular areas, often but not consistently, are 'benign-looking' in growths of low malignancy, but cells of distinctly sarcomatous character may be found in clumps and patches. Osteogenic activity is a basic element; variation from regular lamellar arrangement to irregular spiculation, as well as in the degree of solidity of bony replacement, is common. Some areas, and some tumours, may be so extensively ossified as to hide evidence of stroma cells. Areas of cartilage show similar ranges of cellular type, from differentiated and normal-looking cells to those with atypical active proliferation.

The wide scope of deviation of cytological composition makes the interpretation of limited biopsy material problematical. A 'lucky' snip or core of tissue may show sarcoma cells, but more often the material yields benign pictures. Accurate diagnosis usually demands examination of multiple sections from different parts of the tumour, a procedure which is often only performed when there is a 'recurrence'.

DIFFERENTIAL DIAGNOSIS

The distinction from conventional osteogenic sarcoma has already been noted. The following conditions also raise problems of differentiation:—

Myositis Ossificans

The main points of differentiation are listed in *Table XXVI*, p. 65.

Osteochondroma

Diagnosis problems may arise in regard to the solitary exostosis when it has a broad, sessile base of attachment. However, the radiograph usually demonstrates, albeit irregularly, continuity of cortical and spongy elements of the exostosis with similar elements of parent bone; and there is a lack of involvement of the related cortex which, in the case of juxtacortical osteogenic sarcoma, is a prominent feature.

The cartilage cap of the exostosis characterizes it, and there is no comparable complete cap in the sarcoma. The cytological components, especially the absence or presence of sarcomatous stroma cells, usually clinch the diagnosis.

TREATMENT AND PROGNOSIS

The prognosis has been discussed in the introductory section. Notwithstanding the relatively good outlook because of slow growth in most cases, the treatment of choice is amputation when first diagnosed. Not infrequently local extirpation is the first measure and then the usual sequel of recurrence presents for treatment. Here an even more emphatic decision for amputation is appropriate.

Table XXVI.—DIFFERENTIATION BETWEEN
JUXTACORTICAL OSTEOGENIC SARCOMA AND MYOSITIS OSSIFICANS

	JUXTACORTICAL OSTEOGENIC SARCOMA	MYOSITIS OSSIFICANS
History of trauma .	Seldom, and then ill-defined	Common: usually severe and diagnosed at the time
Post-traumatic evolution	Not traceable as a sequel	Progression of stages usually obvious
Growth of tumour .	Slow but continuous	Finite. Area of ossification becomes stabilized in about 10 weeks
Density of shadow .	Dense	Usually less dense than adjacent cortex
Shape of shadow .	Rounded and massive	Often triangular and laminated; roughly parallel to long axis of bone
Tumour shadow relation to cortex	Continuous at some part	Entirely or almost separate in at least one view
Involvement of cortex	Present	Underlying bone not involved
Relation to surrounding tissues	Invasion may occur	Invariably clearly separated
Histology . . .	Variegated picture with some sarcoma cells	Innocent structure after full development

SARCOMA IN IRRADIATED BONE

Ionizing radiation of bone occurs with external application of X-rays and radium, and from ingested, inhaled, or injected radioactive substances which are stored within bones.

EXTERNAL RADIATION

Bone sarcomata are rare, but there are reports (Cahan, Woodard, Higinbotham, Stewart, and Coley, 1948; Sabanas, Dahlin, Childs, and Ivins, 1956) strongly inculpating therapeutic irradiation as the primary cause. Coley (1960) collected 86 cases reported in the literature up to 1957. Therapy by gamma or roentgen ray had been given in these cases for a variety of conditions: simple tumours and inflammations of soft and bony tissues, dermatoses, prophylaxis following orchidectomy for testicular seminomata, joint tuberculosis, etc. Sarcomata seem to arise after heavy or prolonged dosage.

The early effects of ionizing radiation are aseptic necrosis followed by repair. Where the overlying tissue (especially the mucosa of the mouth and nose) is also injured and breached, osteomyelitis is a common complication. Healing of radiation osteitis is irregular, with patchy areas of sclerosis enclosing areas of persistent necrosis. Such loculi may contain fibrous tissue in varying degrees of degeneration and maturity; and it seems feasible that cells from this tissue provide the histogenic source of sarcoma. The latent interval before the diagnosis of sarcoma varies from about 5 to 20 years.

Several classes of bone tumours are treated by irradiation. The benign lesions, chondroblastoma, monostotic fibrous dysplasia, and solitary bone cyst, do not of themselves have a propensity to malignant transformation. Thus, post-irradiation sarcoma in these tumours is most probably due to the treatment. Giant-cell tumours are in another category in view of the 'spontaneous' change to overt sarcoma in a certain number of cases. But here, too, there is evidence pointing to the culpability of irradiation. 'Spontaneous' change takes place progressively, whereas irradiation-induced sarcoma usually appears as a new event after a quiet period of some years during which the giant-cell tumour seems to have been cured. In a series of 10 frankly sarcomatous giant-cell tumours, Pan, Dahlin, Lipscomb, and Barnatz (1964) report that 9 had received radiation therapy before the cytological transformation.

DIAL PAINTER'S BONE SARCOMA

In 1931 Martland drew attention to the development of bone sarcoma in girls employed as dial painters. The paint, a phosphorescent zinc sulphide, contains radioactive substances, mainly radium and mesothorium. It is applied by a thin brush. In order to give the brush a fine point, the working girl licks it and so repeatedly swallows minute quantities of radioactive material. It is estimated that about 5 mg. was so ingested in a period of 6 months. Much of the material is stored in bones, being concentrated in sites of osseous tissue formation at zones of growth or maintenance. It may be mobilized from one site and redistributed to another when there is an alteration of bone activity.

Within 2–5 years evidence of radium/mesothorium poisoning and radiation osteitis was frequently found. In 1952 Aub, Evans, Hempelmann, and Martland described the later changes. Areas of bone destruction are replaced by fibrous tissues, which show as irregular patches of rarefaction set in dense zones of sclerotic bone. The bones are more vulnerable to trauma and pathological fractures are common. This often appears to initiate, or release and bring to light, frank neoplastic change.

In about 20 per cent of cases (a percentage that is increasing with the passage of time), after a latent interval of an average of 17 years, sarcomata developed. The tumours were either osteogenic sarcomata or fibrosarcomata and their principal sites were in the lower femoral and upper tibial metaphysis (*Fig.* 10).

INTERNAL 'THERAPEUTIC' RADIOACTIVE DRUGS

Aub and others (1952) include in their paper a report of 5 instances of bone sarcoma following oral or intravenous radium and/or mesothorium, given therapeutically for hypertension, arthritis, or anaemia. Looney, Hasterlik, Brues, and Skirmont (1955) reported similar cases. The sequelae and time relationships are much the same as in the luminous dial painters.

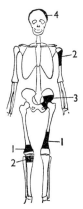

Fig. 10.—Common sites of dial painter's osteogenic sarcoma (right) and of sarcomatous change in Paget's disease (left), where the femur and humerus account for 50 per cent, the pelvis for 20 per cent, and the skull for 10 per cent.

NUCLEAR HAZARDS

Radioactive fission products, particularly strontium 90, are strongly suspect as potential sarcoma-inducing agents. In the experimental animal this isotope is readily absorbed and stored in bone, with consequent bone sarcoma formation.

SARCOMA IN PAGET'S DISEASE

The incidence of Paget's disease is remarkably high. Schmorl (1932) found it in 3·5 per cent of males and 2·5 per cent of females in an unselected series of over 4600 autopsies. Collins (1956) recorded a similar incidence. The tendency for supervention of sarcoma is estimated by some authorities as about 10 per cent in diffuse or polyostotic Paget's disease, and 0·2 per cent in the monostotic forms. However, other observers place the figures at a higher level. Coley (1960) records an incidence of 21·9 per cent in a series of 228 cases. In this group males were affected by sarcoma almost twice as often as females, and the peak age of occurrence was from 50 to 70 years. The commonest sites affected were the femur and the humerus, accounting for 50 per cent; 20 per cent were discovered in pelvic bones, and 10 per cent in the skull (*Fig.* 10).

The clinical heralds of tumour formation are pain and swelling, or sudden alteration and enlargement of a previous known deformity, which may have undergone very gradual change for many years.

Radiographically, the generally thickened bone of Paget's disease shows an area of irregular rarefaction and tumefaction. Less commonly, areas of increased ossification and density appear. Occasionally sarcomatous lesions appear in multiple foci in one or more bones.

Osteogenic activity is usually minimal and may be absent: osteolysis is common, with the formation of haemorrhagic and degenerative cysts.

67

Histological examination may show fibrosarcoma, which occurs in different grades of differentiation and anaplasia. Some lesions show giant-cell tumour characters of the more malignant type. Many tumours show some degree of osteoid or osseous formation and a few are heavily osteogenic.

The prognosis is poor. With few exceptions, sarcomata superimposed upon Paget's disease cause death within 6–12 months. The few exceptions to this gloomy picture are those who have had amputations at an early stage of malignancy.

SARCOMA IN FIBROUS DYSPLASIA AND GIANT-CELL TUMOUR

Osteogenic sarcomata occur but are uncommon in both monostotic and polyostotic fibrous dysplasia. Two references to the literature are noted in the section on Fibrogenic Bone Tumours.

In a later section the supervention of frank sarcoma upon giant-cell tumours is noted. Its incidence is variously estimated at from 10 to 15 per cent. Examples of lung metastases of typical giant-cell tumour components are rare; the usual pulmonary secondaries from primary giant-cell tumours of bone are frank spindle-cell sarcomata.

NEOPLASM IN OSTEOMYELITIS

Chronic osteomyelitis with persistent sinuses discharging onto the skin is still a fairly common condition among communities distant from, or fearful of, adequate medical care. The proportion developing malignant neoplastic change is generally small, but tends to increase with increasing duration of the osteomyelitis. In a series of 9 personally observed cases, the diagnosis of neoplastic supervention was made from 16 years to about 42 years after the onset of the inflammatory condition. The commonest site of neoplasia was the tibia, which accounted for 6 cases. There was one each in the femur, the iliac crest, and the radius.

In all 9 cases the lesion was a squamous-cell carcinoma, presumably originating from chronically inflamed skin epithelium near the orifice of the sinus, or from an epithelized portion of the sinus track. Bone tissue in all cases was invaded by carcinoma cells.

While no case of sarcomatous transformation was observed in this series, this form of malignancy does occasionally occur (Jaffe, 1958).

EXTRA-SKELETAL OSTEOGENIC SARCOMA

This rare lesion may arise in foci of extraskeletal ossification. Occasionally the tumour is a soft-tissue fibrosarcoma which either develops the capacity for osteoblastic activity or is passively ossified as a result of appropriate environmental conditions. In 1956 Fine and Stout recorded 46 cases of sarcoma developing in association with extra-skeletal bone formation.

REFERENCES

AUB, J. C., EVANS, R. D., HEMPELMANN, L. H., and MARTLAND, H. S. (1952), 'The Late Effects of Internally-deposited Radioactive Materials in Man', *Medicine*, **31**, 221.
CAHAN, W. G., WOODARD, H. Q., HIGINBOTHAM, N. L., STEWART, F. W., and COLEY, B. L. (1948), 'Sarcoma Arising in Irradiated Bone. Report of 11 Cases', *Cancer*, **1**, 3.

COLEY, B. L. (1960), *Neoplasms of Bone*, 2nd ed. New York: Hoeber.

COLLINS, D. H. (1956), 'Paget's Disease of Bone: Incidence and Subclinical Forms', *Lancet*, **2**, 51.

DWINNELL, L. A., DAHLIN, D. C., and GHORMLEY, R. K. (1954), 'Parosteal (Juxtacortical) Osteogenic Sarcoma', *J. Bone Jt Surg.*, **36A**, 732.

FINE, G., and STOUT, A. P. (1956), 'Osteogenic Sarcoma of the Extraskeletal Soft Tissues', *Cancer*, **9**, 1027.

GESCHICKTER, C. F., and COPELAND, M. M. (1951), 'Parosteal Osteoma of Bone: A New Entity', *Ann. Surg.*, **133**, 790.

JAFFE, H. L. (1958), *Tumors and Tumorous Conditions of the Bones and Joints*. Philadelphia: Lea & Febiger.

— — and SELIN, G. (1951), 'Tumors of Bones and Joints', *Bull. N.Y. Acad. Med.*, **27**, 165.

LOONEY, W. B., HASTERLIK, R. J., BRUES, A. M., and SKIRMONT, E. (1955), 'A Clinical Investigation of the Chronic Effects of Radium Salts Administered Therapeutically', *Am. J. Roent.*, **73**, 1006.

MARTLAND, H. S. (1931), 'The Occurrence of Malignancy in Radioactive Persons', *Am. J. Cancer*, **15**, 2435.

PAN, P., DAHLIN, D. C., LIPSCOMB, P. R., and BARNATZ, P. E. (1964), 'Benign Giant Cell Tumour of the Radius with Pulmonary Metastases', *Proc. Staff Meet. Mayo Clin.*, **39**, 344.

SABANAS, A. O., DAHLIN, D. C., CHILDS, D. S., jun., and IVINS, J. C. (1956), 'Postradiation Sarcoma of Bone', *Cancer*, **9**, 528.

SCHMORL, G. (1932), 'Über Osteitis Deformans Paget', *Virchow's Arch. path. Anat. Physiol.*, **288**, 694.

WILLIS, R. A. (1960), *Pathology of Tumours*, 3rd ed. London: Butterworths.

CHAPTER 8

FIBROSARCOMA OF BONE

Primary fibrosarcoma takes origin from endosteal connective tissue and produces only collagen. It exhibits a wide spectrum of malignancy from just beyond the dividing line between it and benign desmoplastic fibroma to marked anaplastic forms.

Secondary fibrosarcomata are those superimposed upon previous bone disease, e.g., Paget's disease.

Direct invasion fibrosarcoma of bone involves bone by extension from adjacent tissues, either periosteum or from soft tissue further removed.

PRIMARY FIBROSARCOMA

INCIDENCE

It constitutes 5·8 per cent of primary malignant tumours of bone in the New York Memorial Hospital series (Coley, 1960), and about 7 per cent of the series of primary malignant bone tumours collected by the Bristol Bone Tumour Registry from 1946 to 1967 (Eyre-Brook and Price, 1969).

AGE

It appears mainly after the age of 30 years. It is rare in children.

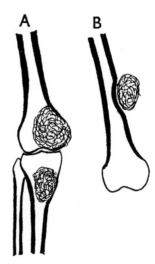

Fig. 11.—**A**, Common sites of primary 'endosteal' fibrosarcoma of bone. In the femur, the epiphysis has been invaded and the cortex penetrated. In the tibia, the cortex has been expanded and thinned in the metaphysial region. **B**, Parosteal sarcoma hollows out adjacent bone, usually its diaphysial portion.

SEX

A number of reports give varying proportions: in total sum, there is no significant difference in sex incidence.

SITE

It usually begins in the medulla, most commonly in a metaphysis of the femur or tibia. In many cases the tumour appears to begin centrally within the bone, but in some a more cortical eccentric zone appears as the original site. It may also involve the epiphysis and can occur in other bones (*Fig.* 11).

CLINICAL PICTURE

Increasingly severe pain is the outstanding feature. It may constitute the sole evidence for a period varying with the aggressiveness of the tumour. The onset may be ascribed to trauma, but this factor probably operates only by calling attention to an already existing tumour. Pathological fractures are not infrequent.

A swelling usually appears some time after the onset of pain, sooner in anaplastic types and later in differentiated tumours. Haematogenous metastases are also usually correlated with the grade of malignancy.

RADIOGRAPHIC PICTURE

The tumour is generally translucent, often with loculation and irregular trabeculation or 'melting-away' of portions of bone affected. Apart from occasional, slight, and then usually late, subperiosteal bone reaction, there is no new bone formation.

The tumour is most extensive in the medulla, but the cortex is almost invariably found to be involved, being eroded and reduced in thickness. Moderate expansion is common and penetration occurs early in undifferentiated lesions. Demarcation is conspicuously absent.

The radiological appearances do not often differentiate the condition from a number of other malignant diseases of bone, but it is helpful in separating benign affections.

MORBID ANATOMY

The mature fibrosarcoma advances very slowly. It is firm and light grey in colour, with areas of whorled, whitish collagen fibres.

Anaplastic lesions are softer, less compact, and whiter. There is more evidence of destruction and erosion without the formation of much collagen. It has usually extended beyond the boundaries of the bone by the time it is removed.

MORBID HISTOLOGY

The mature lesion exhibits spindle-shaped, elongated fibroblasts, often arranged in whorled bundles intermingling with collagen fibres in similar arrangement. The fibroblasts are of uniform size and shape, and, but for the larger, plumper nuclei, the histological picture closely resembles that of the benign desmoplastic fibroma.

Anaplastic fibrosarcomata show pleomorphism, bi- or multinucleate cells, deeply staining nuclei, increased concentration of cell population, and varying numbers of cells undergoing mitosis. Characteristically, fibres are formed to the exclusion of other types of connective-tissue matrix.

Between the extremes of low- and high-grade malignancy described in the foregoing, there is a wide range of intermediate stages. In none of the grades is there any evidence of osteoid or osseous formation, a crucial point of differentiation from osteogenic sarcoma.

DIFFERENTIAL DIAGNOSIS

Desmoplastic Fibroma

The separation of this benign tumour from the well-differentiated fibrosarcoma may pose insoluble issues until time indicates the progress of the lesion. Clinically and radiologically the conditions are often indistinguishable. On microscopy, the desmoplastic fibroma presents a more mature fibrous tissue with a regular cell structure, and an absence of activity and mitoses. Even this appearance may be deceptive because extensive search may reveal the presence of a larger, plumper nucleus to indicate that the lesion has crossed over to the malignant side of the border line.

Fibrous Dysplasia

This may raise difficulties in diagnosis. However, the combined bone destructive and formative elements in the fibrous dysplasia is important evidence as is a high content of alkaline phosphatase by contrast with that in fibrosarcoma where the content is low.

Chondromyxoid Fibroma

Histological examination of some areas of this tumour may give difficulty in diagnosis. Its general character with a nodular pattern, clear definition, and the white zones of chondroid and grey areas of myxoid lobules on its cut surface enable a satisfactory separation from fibrosarcoma to be made. The variety of tissues and the marked range of cytological appearances from different parts of the tumour provide further points of differentiation from fibrosarcoma.

Non-osteogenic Fibroma

Radiologically, this condition is clearly demarcated from unaffected bone by a sclerotic rim, whereas in fibrosarcoma, bony sclerosis is absent. The non-osteogenic fibroma usually presents under the age of 20 years; fibrosarcoma, on the contrary, presents mainly after the age of 30 years.

Histologically, the regular pattern of the arrangement of fibrous tissue without many cells and with slight evidence of activity points to the benign condition.

Osteolytic Osteogenic Sarcoma

This condition exhibits a lower age incidence, viz., under 20 years as against over 30 years in fibrosarcoma, a greater degree of invasive destruction of the cortex without bulging it, and the presence of osteoid and osseous change within the tumour by contrast with its characteristic absence in fibrosarcoma. In addition to these features (see Table XXII, p. 59) Jeffree and Price (1965) have further strengthened the evidence for differentiation by demonstrating that the alkaline phosphatase content of the osteogenic sarcoma is high, whereas it is low in fibrosarcoma.

Treatment and Prognosis

The marked difference in prognosis, ranging from very poor in anaplastic lesions to quite favourable in mature tumours, calls for differences in management. The more malignant tumours require high-level amputation or disarticulation; the less malignant tumours may be locally removed, reserving radical amputation for recurrence if it occurs.

Fibrosarcomata are much less sensitive to radiotherapy than are osteogenic sarcomata; none the less, some beneficial results, both as an adjunct to surgery and as the sole treatment, have been claimed. For those tumours inaccessible to surgery, it remains the main method of treatment.

The prognosis for highly anaplastic lesions is poor, even after extensive ablation. Nearly all cases succumb within a year with widespread pulmonary metastases. The prognosis following radical amputation for intermediate lesions is hopeful. In the Bristol Series (Eyre-Brook and Price, 1969) the 5- and 10-year survival rates are given as 28 and 12 per cent, respectively.

Secondary Fibrosarcoma

Paget's Disease

Fibrosarcomata may be superimposed on Paget's disease. It is commonly held that in most cases of sarcomatous transformation of this disease, the tumour shows evidence of the laying down of osteoid tissue and osseous spicules, and that the tumour is therefore an osteogenic sarcoma. According to this view, in those cases in which only collagen and fibroblasts are found, and therefore fibrosarcoma may be diagnosed, the question of a missed focus of osteogenic activity remains as a shadow of doubt on the diagnosis. Notwithstanding these considerations, Eyre-Brook and Price (1969) report 11 examples of fibrosarcoma following Paget's disease, in all of which cases the pathologists of the Bone Tumour Registry Panel agreed on the diagnosis of non-osteogenic fibrosarcoma.

The survival time for fibrosarcoma superimposed upon Paget's disease is shorter than that for primary fibrosarcoma.

Radiation Osteitis

In radiation osteitis, sarcomatous transformation is more often osteogenic than fibroblastic. This relative incidence holds good whether the radiation is externally applied, as by X-rays, or internally, as by ingested radioactive materials.

Calcified Cartilage Lesions

In their review of 50 cases of fibrosarcoma of bone, Eyre-Brook and Price include 3 cases in which the tumour arose secondarily at the site of an old calcified cartilage lesion.

Parosteal (Periosteal) Fibrosarcoma

The designation is restricted to primary malignant fibroblastic tumours taking origin from the non-bone-forming outer layer of periosteum. It is not a bone sarcoma but it affects bone by pressure or by direct extension of tumour cells. True fibrosarcomata of bone almost invariably begin in the medulla. Occasionally they may, in the early stages, involve mainly one segment of cortex; or the exceptional case (originating in fibrous tissue within cortex or in deep periosteal layers) may also have an eccentric position. Such decentralized localizations were, at one time, referred to as 'periosteal' or 'parosteal' fibrosarcoma, but these terms are best avoided for all endosteal fibrosarcomata, and are preferably used with the limited connotation already noted above.

INCIDENCE

It is a rare tumour.

AGE

The age-group 20 to 40 years is mainly affected.

SEX

It is equally distributed in the sexes.

SITE

Most cases occur next to the diaphyses of the long bones.

CLINICAL PICTURE

A significant number of recorded cases follow distinctly recalled trauma. A lump follows the injury; it may become smaller but it persists. Several years later, because of persistence or increase in size, with or without mild symptoms, it is excised. The excision is usually limited because of the innocent appearances. Then recurrence follows after a year or two. Local excisions and recurrences may occur in sequence on several more occasions until a more radical segmental removal of a block of tissue including the related bone is removed.

RADIOGRAPHIC PICTURE

The tumour shadow is extra-osseous. The cortex of related bone is hollowed or 'spoonerized' by pressure from without, and there is often a rim of sclerosis bordering the hollow (*Fig.* 11 B). Actual invasion of cortex is exceptional. In one personally observed instance, cortical bone was eroded by fibrosarcoma after three previous attempts at surgical removal.

MORBID ANATOMY AND HISTOLOGY

The primary tumour is rounded or ovoid, often appearing to have an enveloping capsule. Bone cortex, if affected, is smoothly hollowed by pressure. In the case quoted of a third recurrence, the cortex was roughened by invading fibrosarcoma tumour.

Histologically, the appearance is almost invariably that of low-grade, spindle-cell fibroblasts.

COURSE AND PROGNOSIS

Progress is slow and this is maintained in early recurrences. Metastases are very rare. Increasing cellularity with plumper nuclei and more pleomorphism may become apparent after several recurrences and are indicative of an evolution to more malignant propensities.

TREATMENT

An initial lesion, and frequently early recurrences, are amenable to local radical removal of a block of tumour and surrounding tissue including bone. Later recurrences, and when invasion of bone has begun, require amputation.

EXTENSION FROM SOFT-TISSUE SARCOMA

The involvement of bone, by pressure or by contiguous extension from a soft-tissue sarcoma, is uncommon. These tumours tend to spread into tissues and tissue planes which offer less resistance to expansive growth and extension, thus usually sparing bone. In regions where the anatomical arrangement restricts soft-tissue extension, e.g., between the metacarpals and the metatarsals, in the carpus and the tarsus, and where interosseous spaces are cramped at the lower end of the forearm and leg, the bones are less infrequently affected.

Of the malignant soft-tissue tumours that invade neighbouring bone, the most common is the fibrosarcoma (Jaffe, 1965). While such sarcomata vary in grade of malignancy, those affecting the limbs tend to be composed of immature cells with invasive properties and recurrence rates of a high order.

The evidence of pressure or invasion from without is usually obvious both radiologically and pathologically. The ovoid, soft-tissue lesion is seen to be depressing cortex into a pond- or spoon-shaped hollow, with a reactive line of sclerosis abutting on the tumour. Intracortical invasion is rare. When it does occur, the probability that the extra-osseous element of the tumour is primary is suggested by its larger size and globular outline, and the reactive features of the invaded bone.

The soft-tissue sarcomata may be of different types and grades of malignancy, thereby influencing the likelihood and extent of bone involvement, and exercising a crucial bearing upon prognosis and treatment. In addition to the anatomical configuration already mentioned, conditions favourable to bone involvement are more apt to be present with deeply placed sarcomata. This is also often correlated with cell type, as the deeper the tumour, the more anaplastic it is. When such a sarcoma is near periosteum, it invades it and reaches and erodes the cortex.

Well-differentiated, soft-tissue fibrosarcomata that involve bone by pressure alone require radical block excision including bone if recurrences are to be prevented. If bone cortex is eroded or penetrated, as may occur after a number of recurrences or with a tumour of undifferentiated cells, amputation is indicated.

It is convenient here to mention several other soft-tissue tumours that may secondarily affect bone: liposarcomata and neoplasms of muscle, cartilage, synovium, and vessels have all figured in reports of occasional bone involvement. They are all much more infrequent causes of such extension than are fibrosarcomata.

REFERENCES

COLEY, B. L. (1960), *Neoplasms of Bone*, 2nd ed. New York: Hoeber.
EYRE-BROOK, A. L., and PRICE, C. H. G. (1969), 'Fibrosarcoma of Bone', *J. Bone Jt Surg.*, **51B**, 20.
JAFFE, H. L. (1965), 'Fibrosarcoma of Bone and Bone Involvement by Direct Extension of Soft-part Sarcoma', in *Tumors of Bone and Soft Tissue*. Chicago: Year Book Medical Publishers.
JEFFREE, G. M., and PRICE, C. H. G. (1965), 'Bone Tumours and their Enzymes', *J. Bone Jt Surg.*, **47B**, 120.

6

CHAPTER 9

GIANT-CELL TUMOUR OR OSTEOCLASTOMA

THE use of these descriptive titles has become restricted to a relatively small group of tumours. The mere presence of multinucleated giant cells does not put a tumour into this group. The definition currently widely accepted is that propounded by Jaffe, Lichtenstein, and Portis in 1940, and with more emphatic clarity by Jaffe in 1953. The definition is based upon the total gross and microscopic patterns, and these are detailed under their respective heads.

The fact that the tumour may recur and occasionally metastasize places it in the malignant class notwithstanding the minor grade of aggression that is commonly exhibited and the benign appearances of the cellular constituents.

INCIDENCE

It is not common. The National Cancer Institute lists it at 5 per cent of all primary malignant tumours of bone.

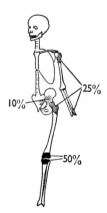

Fig. 12.—Common sites and relative incidence of giant-cell tumour.

AGE

Most cases arise during early adult life, especially from 20 to 40 years; it is uncommon under 20 years and exceptional in childhood.

SEX

In most reported series, females are more often affected.

SITE

The ends of long bones are most commonly involved. The lower femur and upper tibia contribute about half the cases; and the upper femur, lower radius, and upper humerus provide a further quarter to a third (*Fig.* 12).

In long bones the lesion begins in the epiphysis and extends to the metaphysis.

HISTOGENESIS

This is an unsettled question. There are three main contending theories. Konjetzny (1937), among others, regards the giant cells as part of a reparative process reacting to traumatic haemorrhage and granulation-tissue formation. However, a number of factors are not satisfactorily explained on this basis. Traumatic haemorrhage is not specially located at the epiphysial ends of long bones. Trauma is often absent in the history. Further, experimental trauma has not been found to be followed by giant-cell tumours, nor has accidental trauma been connected with this sequel.

The other principal concepts regard it as neoplastic. One, that it arises from osteoclasts, is supported by Geschickter and Copeland (1949) and by Willis (1949) among others. The claim is that the giant cells of the tumour are structurally similar to osteoclasts and that the tumour tissue is similar to that found in other bone-resorptive lesions, e.g., hyperparathyroidism. More recently, in 1961, Schajowicz claimed the demonstration of the presence of the same enzyme systems in giant cells from the tumour and in osteoclasts, so adding support to the osteoclastic theory.

The third theory is advocated by Jaffe and others (1940). They hold that the fundamental cells of the tumour are spindle cells from which giant cells are derived, and that it is therefore incorrect to give the latter cells the emphasis of being the essential neoplastic element. Mary Sherman (1965) supports this view. She finds substantial evidence controverting the view of osteoclast proliferation. Tumour giant cells are often concentrated in tumour tissue where there is no residual bone, and the tumour cells have a different appearance from true active osteoclasts which are found at the periphery of the tumour where bone is undergoing removal. Furthermore, she emphasizes, osteoclasts do not proliferate by division, but they result from fusion of mesenchymal cells.

CLINICAL PICTURE

The primary lesion is almost invariably monostotic. It is usually well advanced by the time when a dull, inconstant pain draws attention to it. Not infrequently the pain and the disability of a pathological fracture are the first subjective evidence, and trauma may feature in the story.

Swelling may sometimes be noted before pain. It is tender, the overlying skin becomes reddish and warm, the veins may become prominent, and 'eggshell crackling' may be elicited in large tumours.

Blood chemistry is not altered.

RADIOGRAPHIC PICTURE

The characteristic involvement of the epiphysial end of the bone with extension to the adjacent metaphysis is shown. The tumour is usually somewhat eccentric, with bulging cortex and, quite often, with bulging of the articular surface on one side.

The general shadow of the tumour is translucent, the cortex being conspicuously thinned. New bone formation is absent or minimal. The cortical shell may be eroded and show defects on roentgen plates; but demarcation is the more usual finding.

The translucency varies in different parts of the same tumour. In a number of cases, but not with any degree of constancy, trabeculation with a soap-bubble appearance is present.

MORBID ANATOMY

Except in very advanced lesions, the tumour is encompassed by a thin shell of bone on its expanded aspect and is limited on its bony side by a distinct layer. Within the tumour there is evidence that bone has been destroyed and removed. The tumour tissue at early stages is solid, soft, friable, fleshy, and red-brown in colour. Later there are greyish areas of collagen and fibrous tissue replacement. Haemorrhages and necrotic degenerations occur and may leave cystic spaces.

MORBID HISTOLOGY

The areas that have not undergone degenerative or collagenous change present the essential tumour pattern. Round to oval, plump stromal cells occupy most of the field, with little intercellular substance between them. The cells have a fairly uniform size, shape, and internal structure. Scattered among them, in parts in more concentrated numbers, are large multinucleated giant cells. Their nuclei resemble those of the stromal cells, suggesting giant-cell development by fusion of many single cells of the stroma.

The density of cellular elements varies. Close crowding intimates great activity and the likelihood of more frank malignancy. Fewer cells, particularly in association with marked fibrotic elements, suggest relatively greater benignancy. Occasionally a group of cells within the tumour is clearly sarcomatous and the course of the tumour is one of rapid local growth and early metastatic spread.

Vascular spaces are prominent. They appear to be lined by the typical stromal cells.

Bony tissue in early or mature form is characteristically absent from the tumour. This characteristic is an important differentiating feature from several other neoplastic conditions of bone.

Metastatic lesions in the lungs rarely show a replica of the benign-looking pattern of the bony primary. For the most part, the secondary site exhibits a sarcomatous cytology.

COURSE AND SPREAD

As has been indicated, progress and spread vary. Some authorities maintain that this is correlated with the cytological constitution of the tumour, viz., the looser the stromal cells, the slower the progress and the more exceptional the metastases. When stromal cells are closely packed, local spread is more rapid, recurrences are somewhat more common and metastases are more likely. When there are obvious sarcomatous changes, the course becomes florid.

Most cases remain localized for sufficiently long to make local removal practicable. In spite of this, Jaffe (1958) and Pan, Dahlin, Lipscomb, and Barnatz (1964) report a recurrence rate of 50 per cent or more following surgery. Jaffe further reports that the recurrences tend to present plumper and more tightly packed stromal cells. Local spread may break through the bony shell and lead to invasion of the soft tissues.

Pan and others (1964) estimate the change to frank sarcoma as about 10 per cent. Most of their cases (9 out of 10) had had ionizing radiation therapy before the cytological transformation.

Thomson and Turner-Warwick (1955) and Jaffe (1958) put the metastatic rate at about 15 per cent. In the rare cases (less than 20 are recorded in the literature) of lung metastases of benign-looking cells, it is supposed that they are emboli of plugs of tumour within veins at the site of the primary lesion. Some of these metastatic lesions have been successfully removed with apparently standard postoperative survival periods. Most lung metastases, however, show obvious spindle-cell sarcoma and behave as such.

Differential Diagnosis
Hyperparathyroidism and Healing Granuloma

Haemorrhagic and/or granulomatous conditions may cause confusion because of the presence of giant cells set in a partly organizing haemorrhagic background in association with different degrees of bone destruction. Two conditions particularly pertinent in this regard are hyperparathyroid 'tumours' and healing

Table XXVII.—Differential Diagnosis—Giant-cell Tumour, Hyperparathyroid Tumour, and Healing Granuloma

	GIANT-CELL TUMOUR	HYPERPARATHYROID TUMOUR	HEALING GRANULOMA
Age . .	20–40 years	20–30 years	10–25 years
Site . .	Epiphysis, spreading to metaphysis	Ends of long bones and jaw may bear solitary lesions	Lower or upper jaw
Multiplicity	Almost invariably monostotic	Commonly multiple sites	One focus
Radiology	Large, defined translucency	Translucent, without distinct borders. Trabeculation common	Translucent
Blood chemistry	No change	Serum calcium and alkaline phosphatase raised. Phosphorus low	No change
Histology .	Plump, round-oval stroma cells	Stroma cells fine and delicate. Ossification common	Small spindle cells in haemorrhagic-granulomatous setting. New osteoid often present
	Absence of osteoid and osseous tissue		
	Scattered giant cells. Vascular channels plentiful	Giant cells of smaller size and clumped next haemorrhage	Giant cells as in hyperparathyroidism

granulomata following traumatic fractures. Although hyperparathyroidism usually affects many bones, its main, or even solitary lesion, may be in the jaw or at the end of a long bone. Healing granuloma is mostly found in the jaw bones. The main points of differentiation between giant-cell tumour and these other two conditions are outlined in *Table XXVII*, p. 79.

Non-ossifying Fibroma
See *Table XVIII*, p. 45.

Benign Chondroblastoma and Solitary Enchondroma
The diagnostic similarities and differences are noted under these headings. See *Table VI*, p. 12, *Table VIII*, p. 15, and *Table IX*, p. 16.

Aneurysmal and Solitary Bone Cysts
The aneurysmal variety, with its blood- or fluid-filled multilocular cysts, is usually amenable to differentiation on gross and radiological appearances. The osseous tissue within its cystic walls is important histological evidence as this type of cell does not appear in giant-cell tumours. The main features have been recorded in *Table XVI*, p. 35, in Chapter 3.

The solitary bone cyst is lined by a fibrous sheet and is filled with fluid. Again, although the radiographic picture may raise the issue of a diagnosis of giant-cell tumour, the microscopic findings are decisive.

The age of presentation of a solitary bone cyst, viz., 3–14 years, and its site in the metaphysis of a long bone, are strong diagnostic beacons.

TREATMENT AND PROGNOSIS
Lesions amenable to surgical extirpation are best dealt with in this manner. Inaccessible lesions call for X-ray therapy.

As the tumour is liable to recurrence in somewhat more than half the cases, and as distant metastases occur in about 15 per cent, it must be regarded as malignant. Accordingly, surgery should be as radical as practicable. Complete removal is curative and is the ideal. It is followed by bone-graft replacement where possible and required. Thorough curetting with bone-chip replacement may have to be accepted as an alternative in certain areas, e.g., the lower end of the femur or the upper end of the tibia.

The latter procedure may be combined with, or in some cases replaced by, X-ray therapy. Many good results, with absence of recurrence for many years, have been reported by surgical curetting and/or ionizing radiation. However, it is after these forms of therapy that the reported recurrences do take place. It has already been noted that recurrence after curetting carries a danger of a change of cell form to a more malignant type, viz., to a more crowded population and to somewhat larger, plumper sizes. Reference has also been made to the high proportion of post-irradiation frankly sarcomatous transformations.

Amputation is occasionally required for recurrence, or marked malignancy, or both.

The rare, cytologically innocent pulmonary metastasis is amenable to cure by lobectomy or pneumonectomy.

REFERENCES

GESCHICKTER, C. F., and COPELAND, M. M. (1949), *Tumors of Bone*, 3rd ed. Philadelphia: Lippincott.

JAFFE, H. L. (1953), 'Giant-cell Tumour (Osteoclastoma) of Bone: Its Pathologic Delimitation and the Inherent Clinical Implications', *Ann. R. Coll. Surg.*, **13**, 343.

— — (1958), *Tumors and Tumorous Conditions of the Bones and Joints*. Philadelphia: Lea & Febiger.

— — LICHTENSTEIN, L., and PORTIS, R. B. (1940), 'Giant-cell Tumor of Bone: Its Pathologic Appearance, Grading, Supposed Variants and Treatment', *Archs Path.*, **30**, 933.

KONJETZNY, G. E. (1937), 'Zur Beurteilung der gutartigen Riesenzellengeschwülste der Knochen', *Chir.*, **9**, 245.

PAN, P., DAHLIN, D. C., LIPSCOMB, P. R., and BARNATZ, P. E. (1964), 'Benign Giant Cell Tumor of the Radius with Pulmonary Metastases', *Proc. Staff Meet. Mayo Clin.*, **39**, 344.

SCHAJOWICZ, F. (1961), 'Giant Cell Tumors of Bone (Osteoclastoma). A Pathological and Histochemical Study', *J. Bone Jt Surg.*, **43A**, 1.

SHERMAN, MARY (1965), 'Giant Cell Tumor of Bone', in *Tumors of Bone and Soft Tissue*. Chicago: Year Book Medical Publishers.

THOMSON, A. D., and TURNER-WARWICK, R. T. (1955), 'Skeletal Sarcoma and Giant Cell Tumour', *J. Bone Jt Surg.*, **37B**, 266.

WILLIS, R. A. (1949), 'The Pathology of Osteoclastoma or Giant-cell Tumour of Bone', *Ibid.*, **31B**, 236.

CHAPTER 10

EWING'S SARCOMA

IN 1921, and with further elaboration in 1924, Ewing described and separated into a distinct entity a tumour which he considered to be of vascular, endothelial cell origin. Ewing abstracted the entity from a broad, ill-defined group of so-called round-cell sarcomata of bone. However, some of these tumours have been withdrawn from Ewing's group by subsequent work and have been placed into separate clinicopathological categories. The main example is lymphoma or reticulum-cell sarcoma, which was delimited and given separate status in 1939 by Parker and Jackson. Ideas about Ewing's sarcoma have been influenced by Oberling's concept, expounded in 1928, of the histogenesis from immature mesenchymal reticular cells of bone-marrow.

The issues of histogenesis and nomenclature are still not settled, and the eponymous designation is justified on this account as well as that of common usage and historical title. In the light of current knowledge, Ewing's sarcoma betokens a primary bone sarcoma consisting of primitive, small, rounded cells, and presenting a combination of distinctive clinical and radiological features.

INCIDENCE

It is not common. Dahlin, Coventry, and Scanlon reported in 1961 that it comprised somewhat less than 10 per cent of all osseous primary malignant tumours. The National Cancer Institute puts it at 11·6 per cent, and at the Memorial Center, New York, the figure is 14·5 per cent.

AGE

Most cases occur during the second decade of life, particularly from 10 to 15 years. The condition is exceptional under 5 and over 30 years.

SEX

It is more common in males; some authors put this as high as 2 males : 1 female.

SITE

Dahlin and others report the femur as the most common site and the innominate bone next. Coley (1960) agrees with this order, but Jaffe (1958) finds the reverse, with the innominate bone accounting for about half his cases. *Fig.* 13 represents a compilation from several sources and gives the relative incidence in the main sites.

CLINICAL PICTURE

Pain is the herald symptom. It progresses in severity and persistence with the passage of months after the onset. Usually, it has endured for 3–9 months by the time the patient is brought for medical attention. A near joint may be tender and have restricted movement. Swelling is common, although it is often partly hidden in a deep situation. Tenderness is a marked feature.

A number of cases present an irregular rise of 1 or 2° in bodily temperature, a moderate but definite leucocytosis, and a raised sedimentation rate—features which may strongly suggest a diagnosis of osteomyelitis or other infection. Lichtenstein (1965), among others, has shown a correlation between these features, often augmented by a secondary anaemia, and the severity of malignancy. Such cases of Ewing's sarcoma run a rapid and fulminating course, with early tumour breakthrough into soft tissue, early and heavy metastases, and death within a few months.

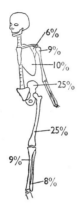

Fig. 13.—Relative incidence of Ewing's sarcoma, in approximate percentages.

RADIOGRAPHIC PICTURE

The tumour shadow is subject to considerable variation. It may present a general translucency with an admixture of patchy or mottled opacities, or opacity may be dominant. All forms are without margins. Medullary involvement is marked and cortical destruction, usually eccentric at an early stage, is notable. Extension of the tumour into extra-osseous tissues is evidenced by cloudy opacity.

Reactive subperiosteal new bone formation may occur but is not particularly frequent. It is, more often than not, irregular. Thus the sign consisting of one or several thin layers of new bone lying parallel to the shaft, and likened to 'onion-peel' or 'plywood', occurs but does not merit the description 'typical' or 'characteristic'. In fact, roentgenographic appearances frequently defy diagnosis or they suggest inflammatory conditions or other malignant tumours. Sherman and Soong (1956), who studied the radiographic appearances of over 100 cases of histologically proven Ewing's sarcomata, concluded that 'the roentgenologist is rarely, if ever, justified in making Ewing's sarcoma his sole diagnosis'.

MORBID ANATOMY

The extent of spread within bone is considerably greater than is suggested by radiography. Spongy bone particularly is widely infiltrated. This holds true, too, for metastatic or multiple primary focal lesions in other bones. Soft tissue is also widely invaded.

The pathological tissue varies in consistency from mushy, semi-liquid to a soft, rubbery but friable quality. Degenerative changes are common, with haemorrhagic and necrotic areas which are most marked in those parts subjected to greatest osteolytic destruction. In other parts the cut surface presents grey-white and glistening rounded masses of tumour.

In innominate bone lesions, tumefaction is usually both external and into the pelvic cavity. Here the tumour mass is often large with compression and distortion of the normal anatomical contents.

The finding of widespread infiltrating lesions in many parts of the skeleton at post-mortem examination is notable and characteristic. Whether these lesions are metastatic from a single primary focus or are multicentric neoplastic responses to a common carcinogenic stimulus is still unsettled.

The lungs and pleurae are commonly, but not invariably, the seats of metastases. Other viscera, e.g., liver, spleen, kidneys, heart, thyroid, etc., may have multiple metastatic deposits.

MORBID HISTOLOGY

In non-haemorrhagic, non-degenerative zones, cells are plentiful and closely packed. They are generally round with large, similarly shaped nuclei containing indistinct, powdery chromatin. The cell outlines are not clearly defined. Degeneration is indicated by fewer cells, by reduction in cytoplasm and nuclear material, by the presence of clear cell borders, and by areas of advancing or complete necrosis which are often surrounded by small round cells giving a pseudo-rosette pattern. Inflammatory reaction, in the form of polymorphs, may dominate certain areas of degeneration.

In Ewing's original description special emphasis was given to the finding of a perivascular or perithelial collar-like arrangement of small round cells. In part it was this appearance that suggested the origin from endothelial cells. However, the advent of small round cells has been shown to be part of the evolution of degeneration; and Jaffe (1958) has emphasized that the perivascular arrangement of cells only occurs where there is haemorrhage and consequent capillary invasion and, further, that the tumour cells do not line the vascular spaces.

There is no characteristic pattern of intercellular substance and there is marked variation in the amount of reticulin fibres in different parts of one tumour as well as in different tumours.

DIFFERENTIAL DIAGNOSIS

Osteomyelitis

Osteomyelitis, both pyogenic and granulomatous, is often wrongly diagnosed instead of Ewing's sarcoma and, conversely, osteomyelitis may be falsely diagnosed as the sarcoma. The main similarities and differences are given in *Table XXVIII*, p. 85.

Eosinophilic Granuloma

A number of features may be common to both conditions and so raise problems of differential diagnosis. Some of the main points are listed in *Table XXIX*, p. 86, which underlines the fact that histological examination may provide the only decisive evidence.

Reticulum-cell Sarcoma of Bone

Difficulties in differential diagnosis are highlighted by the fact that some authorities, e.g., Stout (1934), consider the two tumours as variants of one fundamental pathological entity. However, other authorities lay stress on certain distinctions. The main features are noted in *Table XXX*, p. 86.

Table XXVIII.—Similarities and Differences—Ewing's Sarcoma
AND Osteomyelitis

	EWING'S SARCOMA	OSTEOMYELITIS
Pain . .	Becomes persistent	Similar
Tenderness .	Common	Similar
Fever . .	Not infrequent; mild	Frequent; usually higher
Leucocytosis .	Not infrequent	Frequent
Sedimentation rate	Increased	Similar
Radiography .	May simulate osteomyelitis	May be confused
Operative exploration	May not be characteristic; and appearance simulates osteomyelitis	May be confused
Histology .	Some zones of polymorph infiltration but otherwise cytology is differentiating	Cytology is crucial in differentiation

Osteogenic Sarcoma

The main clue to diagnosis may be the cytological characters. The points are noted in *Table XXXI*, p. 87.

Metastatic Neuroblastoma

Confusion may arise on histological examination. The differentiating features are listed in *Table XXXII*, p. 87.

PROGNOSIS

The disease is virtually always mortal. Fulminating cases terminate within 6 months or so from the onset of symptoms. Less rapidly advancing cases may continue life for about 2 years. Deep therapy may prolong life for an additional year or two.

TREATMENT

Radiation therapy is somewhat better than radical amputation, as the latter adds the pain, anxieties, and disabilities of the operation to the symptoms of the disease, and carries little or no hope of cure. Radiation has greater palliative effects and there are a few 'cures' reported. High dosage and wide application, at least to the whole extent of the bone affected, are required.

Table XXIX.—DIFFERENTIAL DIAGNOSIS—EWING'S SARCOMA AND
EOSINOPHILIC GRANULOMA

	EWING'S SARCOMA	EOSINOPHILIC GRANULOMA
Age . .	Peak 10–20 years	Similar
Multiple lesions	Probably invariable	About half the cases have multiple lesions
Symptoms .	Pain, tenderness, swelling	Often similar, but pain usually less intense
Leucocytosis .	Not uncommon	Usual, and associated with eosinophilia
Radiography .	Demarcation absent	Demarcation usual, but sometimes absent
	Cortex penetrated. Periosteal new bone sometimes	Cortical penetration is unusual, but may occur in association with periosteal new bone
Reaction to radiation therapy	Temporary improvement	Improvement common
Histology .	Variegated picture of plump rounded cells, small round cells, and other changes accompanying degeneration	Dominant cells are histiocytes and eosinophils

Table XXX.—DIFFERENTIAL DIAGNOSIS—EWING'S SARCOMA AND
RETICULUM-CELL SARCOMA OF BONE

	EWING'S SARCOMA	RETICULUM-CELL SARCOMA
Age . .	Peak 10–20 years	Most above 20 years
No. of lesions .	Multiple	Usually limited to one bone; and metastases are late
Prognosis .	Very poor	Relatively much better
Radiography .	Pictures may be similar	—
Histology .	Round cells, with greater degree of uniformity. Cytoplasm poor and vacuolated. Reticulin often sparse or absent	Round cells but with larger nuclei. More variation of structure. Cytoplasm more defined. Present around and between cells
Cure . .	Doubtful if it ever occurs	Probably 20–25 per cent

Both bone primary lesions and lung metastases are remarkably sensitive to ionizing radiation; bone lesions melt away and, radiographically, normal anatomy may be almost completely restored.

Table XXXI.—Differential Diagnosis—Ewing's Sarcoma and Osteogenic Sarcoma

	Ewing's Sarcoma	Osteogenic Sarcoma
Age . . .	10–20 years	10–20 years
Clinical picture .	May be similar in both	—
Radiography .	Not characteristic	Osteolytic and sclerosing types can be simulated
Histology . .	Characteristic round cell	Essential cell is spindle-shaped stromal cell

Table XXXII.—Differentiation between Ewing's Sarcoma and Neuroblastoma

	Ewing's Sarcoma	Neuroblastoma
Age . .	Peak: 10–20 years Rare under 5 years	Common under 5 years Rare after 10 years
Rosettes of cells	Centrum composed of degenerating cells	Centrum composed of neural fibrils, but may degenerate
Primary . .	In bone	Adrenal or other 'sympathetic' tissue
Skull lesion .	Not common; mainly osteolytic when it occurs	Often orbital region causing proptosis; mainly osteoblastic
Multiple bone lesions	Many bones	One or few. Seldom many
Lymph-nodes .	Very exceptionally affected	Often affected; including nodes related to bone metastases

The apparent remission is of short duration and the tumour reappears all too quickly. Second treatments are seldom as effective and usually within 3–18 months the tumour advances beyond control.

The effects of cytotoxic and other chemical agents have so far been disappointing, but many controlled trials have still to be reported.

REFERENCES

COLEY, B. L. (1960), *Neoplasms of Bone*, 2nd ed. New York: Hoeber.

DAHLIN, D. C., COVENTRY, M. B., and SCANLON, P. W. (1961), 'Ewing's Sarcoma: A Critical Analysis of 165 Cases', *J. Bone Jt Surg.*, **43A**, 185.

EWING, J. (1921), 'Diffuse Endothelioma of Bone', *Proc. N.Y. path. Soc.*, **21**, 17.

— — (1924), 'Further Report on Endothelial Myeloma of Bone', *Ibid.*, **24**, 93.

JAFFE, H. L. (1958), *Tumors and Tumorous Conditions of the Bones and Joints*. Philadelphia: Lea & Febiger.

LICHTENSTEIN, L. (1965), *Bone Tumors*, 3rd ed. St. Louis: Mosby.

OBERLING, C. (1928), 'Les Réticulosarcomes et les Réticuloendotheliosarcomes de la Moelle Osseuse (Sarcomes d'Ewing)', *Bull. Ass. fr. Étude Cancer*, **17**, 259.

PARKER, F., jun., and JACKSON, H., jun. (1939), 'Primary Recticulum Sarcoma of Bone', *Surgery Gynec. Obstet.*, **68**, 45.

SHERMAN, R. S., and SOONG, K. Y. (1956), 'Ewing's Sarcoma: Its Roentgen Classification and Diagnosis', *Radiology*, **66**, 529.

STOUT, A. P. (1934), 'A Discussion of the Pathology and Histogenesis of Ewing's Tumor of Bone Marrow', *Am. J. Roent.*, **50**, 334.

CHAPTER 11

BONE LESIONS IN MALIGNANT NEOPLASMS OF HAEMOPOIETIC TISSUES

THE unsatisfactory state of the classification of malignant conditions of myelo-lympho-reticular tissues reflects the many gaps in our knowledge of the pathology. Confusion is further confounded by the absence of an agreed nosological approach.

Of the conditions that fall into the group of haemopoietic tissue neoplasias, multiple myeloma appears to have a firm basis as a primary bone tumour. Reticulum-cell sarcoma, known also as 'malignant lymphoma of bone', is dealt with as a separate entity, but its status as a lymphoreticular tumour arising specifically and primarily in bone is insecure. In myelocytic leukaemia and chloroma, the evidence suggests a probable primary origin in bone-marrow; but in Hodgkin's disease and lymphosarcoma, with or without lymphocytic leukaemia, the possibility of histogenesis in skeletal structures is remote and is hinted at in a small minority of the bone lesions associated with these conditions.

Haematological manifestations of the various neoplastic diseases are not primary phenomena; they are sequels to the overflow of tumour cells from their site of origin into the blood-stream. When blood examinations reveal the presence of cells in appreciable numbers, the condition is called 'leukaemia'. In the following tentative list of skeletal tumours arising as possible primary sources of haemopoietic and lymphoreticular neoplasia (*Table XXXIII*), the type of leukaemic state that may occur is included.

Table XXXIII.—SKELETAL LESIONS ASSOCIATED WITH HAEMOPOIETIC AND RETICULAR SYSTEM MALIGNANCY

LOCALIZED BONE TUMOUR	GENERALIZED 'HAEMIC' STATE	HISTOGENESIS	PRIMARY IN BONE
Myeloma . .	Plasmocytic leukaemia	Plasma cells in bone-marrow	Strongly probable
Reticulum-cell sarcoma or malignant lymphoma	Monocytic leukaemia	Can arise from mesenchymal cells in bone-marrow	Possible
Red marrow infiltration	Myelocytic, or granulocytic, leukaemia	Myelocyte in bone-marrow	Probable
Hodgkin's disease .	—	Exceptionally from reticulum cells in bone-marrow	Possible on occasions
Lymphosarcomatous infiltration	Lymphocytic leukaemia	Lymphoreticular tissues (extra-osseous)	Unlikely

MULTIPLE MYELOMA

This tumour arises in bone-marrow and tends to spread widely to affect many bones. Its cells show the characters of plasma cells in different stages of development and the tumour is often called a 'plasma-cell myeloma'. It is frequently accompanied by a derangement of serum protein.

INCIDENCE

Dahlin (1965) reports that it is the most common of the primary malignancies of bone at the Mayo Clinic. At the New York Memorial Center (Coley, 1960) it accounts for 17 per cent of primary malignant tumours, and comes third in the list of incidence. By comparison with leukaemia generally, myeloma presents in a ratio from 1 : 5 to 1 : 9 (Pinniger, 1958).

AGE

About 75 per cent occur between 40 and 70 years. It is rare under 30 years.

SEX

It is more common in males. Some authors give the ratio as high as 2 : 1, but generally most records show a slight difference.

HISTOGENESIS

The tumour arises from primitive marrow cells.

CLINICAL PICTURE

Pain, of mild and not specifically localized character, is often the sole initial symptom for weeks or months. After a time weakness and anaemia become manifest and the pain may increase in severity and focal sharpness. A more superficial bone may develop an obvious swelling.

Hypercalcaemia may manifest by anorexia, nausea, and vomiting, muscular weakness, mental aberration, and loss of consciousness. There may also be evidence of calculus formation in the urinary tract, perhaps most commonly in the kidney or pelvis.

Oliguria indicates involvement of renal tubules and often portends a fatal end with uraemia.

Bone-marrow

Slides prepared from punctures are important diagnostic guides. An increased percentage of 10 or more in the plasma-cell ratio is strong evidence of multiple myeloma; a count under 10 per cent is not so definite because it may be caused by other conditions.

Blood-picture

Anaemia is marked in about half the cases but because the other half does not exhibit this, it is not a *sine qua non* of the diagnosis.

One or several plasma cells may be found in a blood smear; this is a suspicious sign. Occasionally plasma cells comprise a high proportion of the white cells, the total count of which is then usually high. This is a variant of the condition and is known as plasma-cell or plasmocytic leukaemia.

Serum Calcium

This is often raised when there is extensive bone destruction. Serum alkaline phosphatase is usually normal and inorganic phosphate is commonly raised.

Serum Protein

This is commonly found to be abnormal. It is generally elevated and the albumin: globulin ratio is reversed because of the marked rise in globulins. Among these, the Bence-Jones protein is a frequent component.

Sedimentation Rate

This is often raised.

Bence-Jones Protein in Urine

This is frequently, but not invariably, found. It may also vary from time to time in one patient. Its presence is a strong diagnostic criterion.

RADIOGRAPHIC PICTURE

Before the advent of destruction of bone, X-rays may not reveal any changes, notwithstanding the presence of extensive infiltration. When bone destruction is present, rarefaction, thinning of the cortex on all sides, and varying sizes of punched-out, demarcated translucencies are the characteristic shadows. The last of these evidences may not be present. Expansion of bones is not infrequent, being found especially in the ribs.

MORBID ANATOMY

The condition may, clinically and radiologically, remain localized to one bone for some months, or even a year or two, before becoming manifest in other parts of the skeleton. It would appear that a true 'solitary myeloma' is rare. In most cases of supposed monostotic tumour, the condition is probably present, although hidden, in other bones.

Manifest multiple lesions are more usual. Large numbers of grey or plum-coloured nodules present in the red marrow. The nodules are probably multicentric primary lesions rather than metastases from one focus. The extent of bony change varies in different situations and in different cases. Gross examination may not show noticeable alteration of medullary architecture, despite the presence of diffuse, grey-white, tumour-cell infiltration. All grades between this extreme and marked osteolytic destruction of spongy and cortical bone occur. The tumour mass may grow into the surrounding soft tissue.

Exceptionally, myelomata arise as extramedullary tumours. Most cases have been reported in the mouth or the upper respiratory tract. The condition is relatively benign, but those tumours that do recur after excision tend to progress to the more typical skeletal myelomatosis.

MORBID HISTOLOGY

Different stages of maturity of the plasma cell constitute the essential elements. In some, mature plasma cells predominate, i.e., the type known as 'plasma-cell

7   91

myeloma' or 'plasmocytoma', and is probably the least rapidly advancing of the different lesions. More primitive cells, probably myeloblasts, with pleomorphism and generally larger size, with irregular, more deeply staining nuclear material and a number of binucleate and multinucleate varieties, represent more malignant lesions. Many lesions show a mixed cytological pattern.

SPREAD

It has already been indicated that multiple bone lesions may represent multicentric sites of tumour formation and not metastatic spread. However, involvement of soft tissues does seem to be due to haematogenous and/or lymphatic spread. Nodules of tumour tissue are not uncommon in lymph-glands, spleen, and liver.

Although the kidney is not a site of tumour spread, it is subject to pathological disturbance, probably as a result of the associated upset in serum protein. The 'myeloma kidney' has been described by Mallory (1939), among others. The characteristic finding is plugging of many tubules by a protein material.

The high serum calcium, as in cases of hyperparathyroidism, may lead to the formation of renal calcification and calculi.

DIFFERENTIAL DIAGNOSIS

Hyperparathyroidism

The main points are listed in *Table XXXIV*.

Table XXXIV.—DIFFERENTIAL DIAGNOSIS—MYELOMATOSIS AND HYPERPARATHYROIDISM

	MYELOMATOSIS	HYPERPARATHYROIDISM
Radiography .	Diffuse rarefaction may occur without punched-out areas	Diffuse rarefaction may be similar, and punched-out 'cysts' may appear
Serum calcium .	Hypercalcaemia common	Hypercalcaemia common
Renal calculi .	Common	Common
Serum albumin .	Reversed ratio	Unaffected ratio
Bence-Jones proteinuria	Often present	Absent
Sternal marrow .	Typical plasma-cell picture: diagnostic	Absent

Metastatic Carcinoma

Metastases of osteolytic cancer may be widespread in the skeletal system and present a roentgenographic picture indistinguishable from that of myelomatosis, thus creating problems in the diagnosis when the primary cancer is occult. The main points of similarity and difference are listed in *Table XXXV*.

Table XXXV.—DIFFERENTIAL DIAGNOSIS—MYELOMATOSIS AND METASTATIC OSTEOLYTIC CARCINOMA

	MYELOMATOSIS	METASTATIC CARCINOMA
Age . . .	Mainly 40–70 years	Similar
Radiography .	General irregular rarefaction	Similar: may present punched-out lysed areas
Anaemia . .	Frequent	Common
Serum calcium .	Hypercalcaemia	May also occur
Serum protein .	Hyperglobulinaemia	Not so affected
Bence-Jones proteinuria	Often present	Absent
Sternal marrow .	Usually characteristic and diagnostic	No changes similar to myeloma

PROGNOSIS

It is doubtful whether any form of treatment stays the progress of the disease. In the generalized form, death is almost invariable within a period of a few months to about 3 years. In solitary lesions, the patient may survive for 10 years or more.

TREATMENT

Symptomatic treatment is frequently demanded. Pathological fractures may call for local treatment; anaemia for blood transfusion; hypercalcaemia for prednisone or inorganic phosphate; bacterial infection for antibiotics; uraemia for intravenous and other appropriate therapy; and pain for sedation and palliative radiation therapy.

Irradiation has long been standard as a definitive and beneficial, if short-lived, form of therapy. Apart from relieving pain, it often leads to resolution of the lesions, particularly when the treatment is first applied. However, as other sites of the general condition make their appearance or recurrences occur, they become progressively less responsive to irradiation. Moreover, the sequel of pancytopenia following repeated doses of radiation therapy becomes a disadvantage.

Kyle, Maldonado, and Bayrd (1968) criticize radiotherapy for multiple myeloma from this point of view. Whilst they concede that the main indication for radiotherapy is the supposedly solitary lesion, they hold that the disease is usually obviously diffuse at an early clinical stage and that it is more responsive to chemotherapy than it is to radiotherapy. Therefore radiotherapy should not be allowed to spoil the possibility of using chemotherapy which could be contra-indicated by leucopenia.

These authors present details of the use of the main chemical agents at present in common use, namely, L-phenylalanine mustard (melphalan) and cyclophos-phamide. Other chemical agents are being tried, and urethane, once popular, has been discarded as a treatment.

Reticulum-cell Sarcoma or Malignant Lymphoma of Bone

This condition was first distinguished and separated from Ewing's sarcoma in 1939 by Parker and Jackson. They drew attention to the existence of a primary lymphoma in bone and they coined the term 'reticulum-cell sarcoma' as its designation. As has been mentioned in the preceding chapter on Ewing's sarcoma, some authorities deny the validity of the idea that it is a separate entity and regard it as a variant of Ewing's sarcoma. However, in the state of present knowledge, certain differences appear to be sufficiently noteworthy to vindicate separate classification. These differences are summarized in *Table XXX*, p. 86.

Doubt has also been raised whether the lymphoma is ever primarily and exclusively a bone tumour. It is argued that the condition may be clinically dominant in bone, but the underlying generalized character of the lymphoma is obscured because it has remained small and occult at its site of initial outbreak, i.e., the lymph-nodes or other lymphoid tissue.

The uncertainty has not been resolved, but collective experience (Francis, Higinbotham, and Coley, 1954) favours the proposition that reticulum-cell sarcoma may, on occasion, be a primary neoplasm of bone.

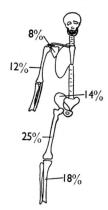

Fig. 14.—Common sites and relative incidence of primary reticulum-cell sarcoma of bone.

Incidence

It is rare. Coley (1960) reports it as constituting 3·2 per cent of all primary malignant bone tumours.

Age

Most cases present from the second to sixth decades, with a peak from 25 to 40 years. It is exceptional under 10 years.

Sex

Males are affected more often, the ratio amounting to 2 : 1.

Site

The main sites and relative incidence, as reported by Francis and others (1954), are indicated in *Fig.* 14.

94

HISTOGENESIS

It probably originates from primitive mesenchyme in bone-marrow.

CLINICAL PICTURE

The main complaint is pain, sometimes associated with swelling. Vertebral lesions cause pain along the course of spinal nerves that are involved by compression. A raised sedimentation is common. Francis and others (1954) stress the apparent good general condition of the patient despite the presence of a large tumour.

RADIOGRAPHIC PICTURE

Irregular zones of rarefaction, often with patchy sclerotic opacities, make up most of the tumour shadow. Parts of the cortex usually show the same effects of tumour invasion. Periosteal new bone, if present, is seldom marked, and there is no new bone formation in extra-osseous extensions. The shaft of long bones is often expanded to a spindle shape.

The picture varies and it is often difficult to differentiate from inflammatory conditions, osteolytic forms of osteogenic sarcoma, metastatic carcinoma, and Ewing's sarcoma.

MORBID ANATOMY

The gross specimen may resemble other tumours, especially Ewing's sarcoma and osteolytic osteogenic sarcoma. Tumour tissue is often soft and friable and, when extensive, necrotic areas are prominent.

Local tumour growth is usually slow; so, too, is distant spread. Regional lymph-nodes may be involved and secondary or additional involvement of other bones also occurs.

MORBID HISTOLOGY

The essential cell, i.e., the reticulum cell, usually contains a single, plump, rounded nucleus which may be folded or indented. The cytoplasm and its boundary appear indistinct. Some cells have prominent double nuclei. Areas of lymphocytes are quite often prominent and in some cases lymphoblasts may be plentiful. Appropriate staining demonstrates the presence of fine reticulum fibres between cells and in broader strands around groups of cells. The picture is essentially the same as that of reticulum-cell sarcomata of lymphoid tissue, and there are no differences between primary and secondary lesions in bone.

DIFFERENTIAL DIAGNOSIS

Ewing's Sarcoma

This has been noted in the preceding chapter in *Table XXX*, p. 86.

'Generalized' Reticulum-cell Sarcoma with Bone Lesion

The distinction between the two conditions depends on a presumption that the reticulum-cell sarcoma is primary in bone when there is no evidence of disease elsewhere or when it precedes the involvement of other tissues and other bony sites by an appreciable period.

The age at which the two conditions present differs to some extent. In the primary bone lesion, half the cases occur under 40 years; in general affections, most cases present above the age of 40 years.

Metastatic Anaplastic Carcinoma

Occasionally, when the primary carcinoma remains hidden, its bony metastasis may present radiological and cytological appearances which closely simulate primary reticulum-cell sarcoma. Diagnosis may require further and wider biopsy material; sometimes it is only defined when the primary focus of carcinoma becomes obvious.

PROGNOSIS

Reticulum-cell sarcoma is often of gradual progress and thus has a much better prognosis than does Ewing's sarcoma. Cures are possible, and the 5-year cure rate may reach 25 per cent.

TREATMENT

Radiation therapy has quite frequently destroyed the local lesion, and this may not be followed by recurrence. However, it is fairly common to find the development of lesions in other bones at a later stage.

Surgical amputation, done in situations amenable to complete extirpation, has also claimed successes.

SECONDARY BONE LESIONS IN RETICULUM-CELL SARCOMA

Reticulum-cell sarcoma, commonly beginning in a lymph-node, tends to spread to other nodes and (in about 15 per cent of cases) to bones, where it may cause the same range of lesions as the 'primary' variety.

Radiation is the treatment of election, with chemotherapy becoming increasingly useful as palliation.

HODGKIN'S DISEASE

Secondary bone involvement is quite common. In cases submitted to autopsy, the incidence is variously reported as, e.g., 60 per cent by Ultmann (1966) and 78 per cent by Steiner (1943). The secondary bone lesion may provide the herald symptom of pain; in Ultmann's 135 cases, 6 per cent began in this way. Many bone lesions remain clinically silent. The commonest bones affected are the vertebral bodies and those of the pelvic ring.

Those who hold that a *primary* Hodgkin's disease of bone does occur apply the following criteria to the diagnosis: The neoplasm appears to begin in a bone and remains restricted to the bony site for a definite period of time. If lymph-node involvement occurs in the course of the disease, it follows the bone lesion and it arises initially in the regional lymphatic drainage area of the primary site in bone before it spreads more generally. Notwithstanding the exceptional cases that match strictly applied diagnostic criteria, the existence of primary Hodgkin's disease is still in doubt, inasmuch as a hidden primary in lymphoid tissue may exist.

Roentgenologically, there are no typical findings and changes may be absent notwithstanding the presence of infiltrating lesions. Recognition of the condition depends upon microscopic study of biopsy specimens.

LYMPHOSARCOMA AND LYMPHOCYTIC LEUKAEMIA

The terminology used here accords with the thesis that lymphosarcoma is the essential neoplastic condition and that the malignant cells, lymphocytes and/or lymphoblasts, may or may not spill into the blood-stream; if they do, then lymphocytic and lymphoblastic leukaemia appropriately describe such development.

Involvement of bone is common in children but rare in adults. It is found particularly in acute leukaemia of the lymphoblastic cell type. Pain in different bones and joints is the principal clinical indication of bone invasion and it may draw attention to the disease. By contrast with metastases from carcinomata, the bones involved frequently include those of the forearm and the leg. As the pains may shift from one bone or joint to another, and pallor, weakness, and slight fever are common, rheumatic fever and Still's disease are often diagnosed. When the bone pains remain localized, osteomyelitis may be suggested.

Radiographic appearances vary. In children they often provide some indication of the presence of bone involvement. In long bones, particularly about the knee-joint, a band of translucency lying adjacent and parallel to the epiphysial plate is an early sign. Other conditions may also produce the sign, e.g., severe debilitating illness and scurvy. As the bone lesion advances, the zone of translucency grows increasingly into the metaphysis; there may be general rarefaction and/or multiple punched-out holes. Larger osteolytic lesions signify still further pathological progress. Proliferative osteoblastic reactions occur quite frequently and show up as laminated periosteal new bone. Radiologically visible changes in adults are seldom found, even in those cases where bone is involved by lymphosarcomatous infiltration which gives rise to clinical signs.

The diagnosis is often established by the blood-picture. In cases with an 'aleukaemic' blood-picture, a not uncommon feature of an acute lymphoblastic lymphosarcoma in children, sternal-marrow preparations nearly always settle the problems.

The condition is invariably fatal. Some forms of therapy are useful palliatives. Ionizing radiation may give temporary relief; but the current tendency is to use cortisone or ACTH together with different folic acid antimetabolites or cytotoxic agents like nitrogen mustard.

MYELOGENOUS LEUKAEMIA

Myelogenous stem cells, or myeloblasts, giving origin to myelocytes (also known as granulocytes and polymorphonuclear leucocytes) with basophil-, neutrophil-, and eosinophil-staining characters, are situated (during late embryonic and post-natal life) in red bone-marrow. Malignant neoplasms of myelogenous tissue are thus initially and primarily bone-marrow tumours. Whether the neoplasm arises from one bony focus or more diffusely from many fields of red marrow is unsolved. By the time the patient presents for clinical assessment, and more markedly by the time a necropsy examination is done, affection is widespread.

The proliferating malignant cells infiltrate and replace fatty marrow, usually in a diffuse pattern and only exceptionally with the formation of macroscopically roughly defined tumours. Because of the greenish coloration of such localized tumour aggregations, the designation 'chloroma' is used.

Probably as an invariable event, tumour cells from myeloblastic neoplasms of bone overflow into the blood-stream to produce myelogenous leukaemia. This is subdivided into acute and chronic forms.

Acute Myelogenous Leukaemia

This form is not uncommon in children, but is rare in adults. The skeletal manifestations, both clinical and radiological, are similar to those described in acute lymphocytic leukaemia.

Chloromata are most likely to occur in the acute variety. The tumour masses develop especially in or near periosteum, and more often in vertebrae, skull, and ribs than elsewhere. The tumefactions may be conspicuous clinically, and they tend to fill soft-tissue cavities, e.g., the orbit and the paranasal sinuses. Chloromata occasionally arise in extraskeletal tissues, the kidneys being the most frequently reported site.

Chronic Myelogenous Leukaemia

This is the common form of leukaemia in the adult. Its peak incidence falls in the third and fourth decades of life.

Symptoms referable to the skeletal system are unusual, differing in this respect from the symptoms of acute leukaemias. One fairly common and prominent sign is tenderness on pressure over the sternum; when this is associated with a grossly enlarged spleen and a moderately enlarged liver, its diagnostic importance is enhanced. Localized, tender bone swellings are occasional findings.

Notwithstanding the dense infiltration of bone-marrow by neoplastic granulocytic cells, it is unusual to have either medullary or cortical destruction. This explains why radiographic signs of chronic granulocytic leukaemia are exceptional. When such signs are found, the changes are focal rather than diffuse.

REFERENCES

COLEY, B. L. (1960), *Neoplasms of Bone*, 2nd ed. New York: Hoeber.

DAHLIN, D. C. (1965), 'Histogenesis and Classification of Bone Tumors', in *Tumors of Bone and Soft Tissue*. Chicago: Year Book Medical Publishers.

FRANCIS, K. C., HIGINBOTHAM, N. L., and COLEY, B. L. (1954), 'Primary Reticulum Cell Sarcoma of Bone', *Surgery Gynec. Obstet.*, **99**, 142.

KYLE, R. A., MALDONADO, J. E., and BAYRD, E. D. (1968), 'Treatment of Multiple Myeloma', *Proc. Staff Meet. Mayo Clin.*, **43**, 730.

MALLORY, T. B. (1939), 'Case Records of the Massachusetts General Hospital', *New Engl. J. Med.*, **221**, 983.

PARKER, F., jun., and JACKSON, H., jun. (1939), 'Primary Reticulum Cell Sarcoma of Bone', *Surgery Gynec. Obstet.*, **68**, 45.

PINNIGER, J. L. (1958), 'Malignant Tumours of the Bone Marrow and the Spleen', in *Cancer*, Vol. 2 (ed. RAVEN, R. W.) London: Butterworths.

STEINER, P. E. (1943), 'Hodgkin's Disease: The Incidence, Distribution, Nature and Possible Significance of the Lymphogranulomatous Lesions in the Bone Marrow: A Review with Original Data', *Archs Path.*, **36**, 627.

ULTMANN, J. E. (1966), 'Clinical Features and Diagnosis of Hodgkin's Disease', *Cancer*, **19**, 297.

CHAPTER 12

MALIGNANT VASCULAR TUMOURS, ADAMANTINOMA, CHORDOMA

A MISCELLANEOUS group of bone tumours is collected together in this section for convenience. The tumours have no proven aetiological or pathological connexion with one another except for their occurrence in bone.

MALIGNANT VASCULAR TUMOURS OF BONE

Haemangiosarcoma

This tumour arises from endothelial cells or their more primitive forebears; the tumour cells continue the function of forming vessels, albeit in an irregular and disorganized fashion.

INCIDENCE

It is a rare condition.

AGE AND SEX

The paucity of recorded cases renders efforts at appraisal of peak age and sex incidence meaningless.

CLINICAL AND RADIOGRAPHIC PICTURE

Pain and swelling are the main features. Radiographically, marked rarefaction of both medulla and cortex with slight bone expansion may be found.

MORBID ANATOMY

Multiple lesions, probably multicentric primaries, are more common than solitary foci. The tumour tissue is often red-brown and soft and tends to fade into the neighbouring bone.

Haematogenous and lymphatic metastases occur.

MORBID HISTOLOGY

The essential element is the primitive endothelial cell, collections of which occur in clumps and strands, filling most of the background to newly formed vascular channels which are lined by the same type of cell.

The greater the differentiation of cell type, the more marked is the vascular pattern. At the opposite pole, where the cells are primitive and anaplastic, vaso-formative activity may be so immature that little or no lumen is to be seen.

DIFFERENTIAL DIAGNOSIS

The main criterion is the histological picture; but this too may be confused with highly vascular primary sarcomata or metastatic carcinomata. In cases where the cytological pattern defies precise diagnosis, it is pertinent to recall the rarity of angiosarcoma and the relative commonness of the other possibilities.

TREATMENT AND PROGNOSIS

Differentiated lesions are of slow growth and are amenable to cure by complete local surgical eradication. The more malignant types call for radical amputation if they are solitary and still localized. If they are not amenable to surgery, radiation therapy may be of some help, but the prognosis is gloomy.

Kaposi's Sarcoma of Bone

Since 1872, when Moricz Kaposi described the condition as a distinct entity affecting the skin, it has been discovered to affect, and probably to arise from, organs other than the skin. Although there is still uncertainty about its primary origin in bone, a number of examples in which the clinical features are dominantly related to bone and in which the main pathological findings are located in bone suggest the possibility of such an origin.

It is a rare condition in many parts of the world, but it is common in certain regions, e.g., in some areas of the Congo basin the incidence reaches a peak of 12·8 per cent of all cancers in the Negro population, i.e., more than 250 times the incidence in Chicago.

AGE

Peak figures are recorded in the 30–50-year age-group. It also affects children and older ages.

SEX

Males preponderate in a ratio of about 10 : 1.

SITE

It may be found in any bone, but the most commonly affected are the small bones of the hands and feet, followed by the leg and arm bones. This peripheral predilection of bone affection corresponds to the pattern of distribution in the skin, where the disease nearly always begins on the feet and hands and subsequently advances centripetally.

HISTOGENESIS

The cell of origin is still in the realm of controversy. Studies by Becker (1962) of tumour-cell morphology, histochemical and enzyme properties did not lead to any conclusive answer. The following list of cellular origins indicates the range and scope of theories about histogenesis and emphasizes the absence of agreement on the subject:—

Reticulum cells, fibroblasts, primitive mesenchyme, lymphatic vascular endothelium, glomus body, Schwann cells of vascular perithelial tissue, and vascular endothelium.

An unexplained association with tumours of the lymphoma group raises yet other speculative theories. Bluefarb (1957) records the combination of Kaposi's sarcoma with mycosis fungoides, Hodgkin's disease, lymphosarcoma, and lymphatic and myeloid leukaemia, in numbers that are too high to be accepted as chance occurrences. However, any temptation to infer that there is a common or similar basic pathology is blocked by the distinctive histopathology of Kaposi's sarcoma.

CLINICAL PICTURE

Bone involvement is sometimes clinically silent, but it may give rise to pain and disability. Bone may be the predominant site of tumour invasion with, or less often without, skin lesions, but apparently invariably accompanied by tumour invasion of other organs, e.g., the gastro-intestinal tract and abdominal viscera, the urogenital and respiratory tissues, the heart, etc.

RADIOGRAPHIC PICTURE

Analyses and reviews of the findings have been recorded by Davies (1956) and Palmer (1962). The latter reviewed 200 cases.

The affected bones are decalcified; trabecular patterns are 'rubbed out' and the cortex is thinned and often expanded. Clear-cut cysts and erosions, appearing like 'bites' out of the margin of the bone, are additional and striking features.

MORBID ANATOMY AND HISTOLOGY

The formation of neoplastic vascular channels confers a red-brown, and sometimes bluish, hue to the cut section of the tumour mass. The consistency varies from fairly firm elastic to soft pulp, especially when haemorrhagic and necrotic zones are prominent. The spread in bone is usually extensive and is commonly without clear margins.

Murray and Lothe (1962) found that wherever the lesion and at whatever age it occurred, the essential cytological pattern was the same. The basic cells are spindle-shaped with pleomorphic nuclei. Aggregations of cells in irregular bundles and fascicles are arranged in whorled, interweaving, sweeping streams, with reticulin and collagen fibres dividing the currents and tributaries of the streams in diverse patterns. Vasoformative activity varies in quantity and appears as slits or clefts containing blood. These channels are not lined by endothelium.

DIAGNOSIS

The problems arise principally in those geographical areas where the tumour is common. Most bone affections are associated with skin lesions which are, in the main, readily diagnosable. Cases without tell-tale evidence in the skin or other organs depend for their recognition upon the characteristic cytological picture.

PROGNOSIS

Tumour virulence varies from slowly growing, relatively benign types to those of fulminating rapidity. The former are compatible with survival for 20 years or so, and the latter cause death within 6–12 months of diagnosis.

TREATMENT

Cytotoxic agents, particularly when given by intra-arterial perfusion and ionizing radiations, have both been claimed as useful palliatives and as holding promise for prolonging life.

Adamantinoma of the Tibia

A resemblance in the histological picture between this tumour and the adamantinoma of the jaw bone is responsible for its questionable title. In the jaw the tumour is of epithelial origin and it tends to produce tissues similar to those derived from the formed or developing enamel organ. In the tibia (and exceptionally in some other long bones), although the histogenesis may be from epithelial elements, the tumour tissue differs from the lesion of the same name in the jaw.

Incidence

The condition is rare. Coley (1960) records the incidence at the New York Memorial Center as less than 0·5 per cent of all malignant tumours.

Age

The tumour appears mainly during adolescence.

Sex

Males predominate in most recorded series.

Site

All reports indicate a large majority of lesions in the shaft of the tibia. A few other occasional sites are mentioned, e.g., radius, femur, and ulna.

Histogenesis

A number of theories relate the origin to epithelial cells. The original hypothesis was that a displaced dermal cell-rest within bone ultimately differentiated into dental epithelial tissue.

The traumatic theory expounded by Ryrie (1932) supposes that injury causes an implantation of epithelial basal cells into bone, where they grow to produce the tumour.

Changus, Speed, and Stewart (1957) consider the tumour tissue to be pseudo-epithelial, actually derived from vascular endothelium. They use the designation 'angioblastoma' to convey their idea.

Hicks (1954), among others, expounds the thesis of a connective-tissue growth with differentiation towards synovial tissue.

All the theories are subject to serious doubt; none of them satisfactorily explains all the cytological patterns.

Clinical Picture

A swelling is the main reason for bringing the condition to notice. Pain is seldom marked, but if it is, it may point to a pathological fracture.

Trauma is often featured in the history, but the tibia is such a common site for trauma that it would be surprising if injuries were not recalled in the story. It would seem that trauma calls attention to an already existing tumour but that it has a very doubtful status as a causative factor.

Radiographic Picture

In most cases the main lesion is in the diaphysial cortex, which is rarefied, sometimes trabeculated, and almost invariably expanded. Adjacent parts of the cortex are often sclerotic. Radiotranslucency may extend from the cortex into the medulla and across the complete diameter of the shaft of the bone.

Morbid Anatomy

The tumour is usually near the mid-shaft of the tibia, occupying some inches of its length. On section, areas of grey-white tumour tissues are firm and vaguely lobulated; other areas are brown to yellow and are softer. Haemorrhagic and degenerative zones are more common in advanced lesions. The tumour appears well defined and the cortex above and below the portion destroyed by the neoplasms is thickened and dense.

Morbid Histology

The misconception that this tumour of the tibia was a variant of the jaw adamantinoma arose from the appearance of epithelial-like cells arranged in alveolar form, sometimes very similar to the appearance of a rodent cancer; in some cases the squamous-cell character was even more strongly suggested by the formation of cell nests. However, epithelial-like elements may be absent or form only part of a variegated picture. Collagen and connective tissue with spindle cells are often prominent. Vascular clefts and other spaces are common, with lining cells which are more like endothelium and which have been described as angioblasts (*see* Histogenesis).

Course and Spread

Direct spread is generally slow. Most of the occasional exceptions with more rapid spread occur in recurrences following local removal. Lymphatic node involvement in the groin has been noted, but is uncommon. Pulmonary metastases are unpredictable. Some appear within a few years of diagnosis, while other cases continue to live with the local tumour for 15–20 years without any evidence of haematogenous spread.

Treatment and Prognosis

Radical local surgical removal is successful in most early cases. It also succeeds quite often in recurrences after a first operation. Later recurrences, and any hint of a more rapidly progressive type, call for amputation.

Chordoma

A chordoma is a malignant tumour which arises from a remnant of embryonic notochord. It occurs mainly at one or other of the extremities of the notochord, viz. at the base of the skull or the sacrococcygeal region.

Incidence

It is rare. In a series of 413 apparently solitary tumours of the vertebral column, Cohen, Dahlin, and MacCarty (1964) found 72 chordomata, which constituted the most common of the primary tumours of the vertebrae. The sacrococcygeal site is the most frequent, followed by the skull. These two account for about 90 per cent of chordomata.

AGE

The tumour may appear at any age; most present in patients over 50 years old.

SEX

Males are affected more often in a ratio of 2 : 1 or 3 : 1.

CLINICAL PICTURE

Pain is the usual herald. With increase in size, radiating pains become noticeable. Constipation and/or diarrhoea and urinary disturbances, retention or incontinence, are not uncommon. A pelvic mass (or posterior sacral tumour, or both) is usually clinically appreciable. In skull lesions many cranial nerves are likely to be affected. The rate of growth varies. Most are very gradual, but occasionally a more aggressive and relatively rapidly growing tumour occurs.

RADIOGRAPHIC PICTURE

At the base of the skull erosion of the sphenoid is common. Air encephalograms often show upward displacement of the third ventricle and distortion of the aqueduct and the fourth ventricle.

At the lower end of the vertebral column there is irregular destruction and expansion of the sacrum. The tumour mass is cloudy and can be distinguished from normal soft tissue. Opaque media introduced into the urinary bladder and bowel often clearly demonstrate the distortion and displacement of these organs by the tumour.

MORBID ANATOMY

At the base of the skull the tumour is usually small, whereas the sacrococcygeal tumour is large. Direct invasion is typical, but tends to be slow and noticeable over a period of years.

At the cranial site the nodular tumour pushes and then invades the dura ahead of it. With penetration, the brain may be compressed or invaded. Neighbouring bones, e.g., of the nasopharynx and the orbit, are often eroded.

In the pelvis the tumour may grow to the size of a foetal head or greater. Extension, with tumefaction on the surface, may occur into the buttocks or posterior to the sacrum. The sacrum and the coccyx are often widely eroded and replaced by tumour.

On section, the tumour is irregularly lobulated and has a jelly-like appearance in parts.

Metastases to lymph-nodes and to the liver and the lungs occur. Occasionally secondary deposits are found in bizarre situations. The total incidence of metastases is variously estimated from 4 to 10 per cent.

MORBID HISTOLOGY

The main distinctive features are the presence of intracellular and extracellular mucin, and large physaliphorous cells with well-marked vacuoles. These are the characters of mature cells. They may be sparse and not noticeable in less differentiated lesions. The tissue is then much more cellular with an anaplastic fibrosarcomatous appearance. Epithelial elements of different grades of maturity, from an extreme of anaplastic syncytial cells to tubular structures lined by cuboidal epithelium, may be found.

TREATMENT AND PROGNOSIS

The technical difficulty of complete surgical removal accounts for the frequency of recurrences and the almost invariable progress to ultimate fatality. Repeated partial removal is justifiable, as it delays progress and may save the patient much pain and discomfort.

REFERENCES

BECKER, B. J. P. (1962), 'The Histogenesis of Kaposi's Sarcoma', *Acta Un. int. Cancr.*, **18**, 477.

BLUEFARB, S. M. (1957), *Kaposi's Sarcoma. Multiple Idiopathic Haemorrhagic Sarcoma*. Springfield, Ill.: Thomas.

CHANGUS, G. W., SPEED, J. S., and STEWART, F. W. (1957), 'Malignant Angioblastoma of Bone: A Re-appraisal of Adamantinomas of Long Bones', *Cancer*, **10**, 540.

COHEN, D. M., DAHLIN, D. C., and MACCARTY, C. S. (1964), 'Apparently Solitary Tumors of the Vertebral Column', *Proc. Staff Meet. Mayo Clin.*, **39**, 509.

COLEY, B. L. (1960), *Neoplasms of Bone*, 2nd ed. New York: Hoeber.

DAVIES, A. G. M. (1956), 'Bone Changes in Kaposi's Sarcoma: An Analysis of 15 Cases in Bantu Africans', *J. Fac. Radiol.*, **8**, 32.

HICKS, J. D. (1954), 'Synovial Sarcoma of Tibia', *J. Path. Bact.*, **64**, 151.

KAPOSI, M. (1872), 'Idiopathisches multiples Pigmentsarkom der Haut', *Arch. Derm. Syph.*, **4**, 265.

MURRAY, J. F., and LOTHE, F. (1962), 'The Histopathology of Kaposi's Sarcoma', *Acta Un. int. Cancr.*, **18**, 413.

PALMER, P. E. S. (1962), 'The Radiological Changes of Kaposi's Sarcoma', *Ibid.*, **18**, 400.

RYRIE, B. J. (1932), 'Adamantinoma of the Tibia: Aetiology and Pathogenesis', *Br. med. J.*, **2**, 1000.

CHAPTER 13

METASTATIC CARCINOMA IN BONE

BOTH carcinomata and sarcomata metastasize to bone. Carcinomatous bone metastases are much more common; in fact they outnumber the combined sum of primary and secondary sarcomata of bone. Many tumours of haemopoietic and reticular tissues involve bone, both as primary and as secondary lesions. The latter metastatic bone tumours have been considered in an earlier section.

INCIDENCE

Estimates vary of the proportion of fatal carcinomata in which there are skeletal secondaries. Willis (1941), in a review of 500 consecutive cancer necropsies, found bone metastases in 14 per cent. Abrams, Spiro, and Goldstein (1950) analysed 1000 consecutive autopsies on cases of carcinoma; there were bone metastases in 27 per cent.

Jaffe (1958) draws attention to several possible fallacies in assessing incidence. Many cases are clinically silent and radiologically negative and, if the main emphasis in investigation of metastases is based on clinical indications or on roentgenographic demonstration, the result will fall far short of the true position. Autopsy findings may be inaccurate because of inadequate examination. When such sources of error are eliminated, and with the added factor of longer survival of many carcinoma cases with current forms of therapy, the incidence (according to Jaffe) is in the region of 70 per cent. In ossophile cancers, his estimate is about 85 per cent.

OSSOPHILE CANCERS

This term is used for those primary cancers which are especially prone to metastasize to bone. The principal ossophile cancers affect the breast, prostate, lung, kidney, and thyroid. There is an opposite type of primary cancer (ossophobe) which seldom causes bone secondaries. The outstanding examples are cancers of the skin, the gastro-intestinal tract, and the cervix.

The relative incidence of primary carcinomata giving rise to skeletal deposits is variously reported by different authors. Obviously, the more common tumours will occasion a higher overall percentage of metastases; and although the less prevalent tumours do not contribute a high proportion of the total bony lesions, they may exhibit a high individual proclivity to such activity. Among females about 70 per cent of all bone secondaries come from breast cancers; of all breast cancers, about 20 per cent cause lesions in bone, and in breast cancer cases submitted to autopsy examination, about 66 per cent show metastatic spread to bones. In males, lung and prostatic cancers are the primary sources of about 70–80 per cent of skeletal involvement; and it is estimated that about 20 per cent of all lung cancers, and some 60 per cent of prostatic tumours, affect bone. Whilst adenocarcinoma of the kidney contributes somewhat less than 5 per cent of osseous metastatic cancer, about 50 per cent of renal lesions are implicated in such spread.

SITES OF BONE LESIONS

Copeland (1931) and Fort (1935), using radiological criteria, found the trunk bones and the skull to be the most commonly affected, followed by the upper metaphyses of femur and humerus. The occurrence in more peripheral bones, especially in the arms, hands, legs, and feet, was exceptional.

Pathological investigation suggests a somewhat different order of frequency. *Fig.* 15 is constructed by combining the experience of a number of authorities and the information given in a general discussion on metastatic lesions in bone by a panel under the chairmanship of McGraw (1965).

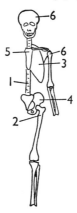

Fig. 15.—Common sites of skeletal metastatic carcinoma. The order of frequency is indicated by numbers.

TIME LAPSE

The bone secondary may be the first indication of the presence of cancer. It is not infrequent that, after the diagnosis of the metastases, the primary eludes discovery for quite a long time and may still remain hidden at autopsy. Occasionally, in differentiated lesions, the cytological picture of the secondary fixes the seat of the primary which, even then, may remain physically occult.

Another important consideration in assessing the time lapse between diagnosis of the primary and advent of the secondary is that the recognition of the latter often depends upon radiographic evidence which may fail to reveal extensive cancerous invasion. It is only when the cancer brings about lytic, sclerotic, or other bone reactions, that radiography is positive. There are many reports of a pathological fracture which brings the condition to attention, the usual sequel being rapid progress of radiographic evidence of malignant advance and destruction.

The span of time between the primary cancer and the secondary deposit in bone is virtually without limit. Examples are on record of breast and thyroid cancers, apparently cured by surgical removal, giving rise to osseous lesions 20–35 years later.

MODE OF SPREAD

The malignant cells reach bone via two routes: the systemic circulation (i.e., by venous route from the primary to the lungs, thence to the left side of the heart and onwards with arterial vessels) or the free communications that exist between systemic veins and the vertebral system of veins (Batson, 1940, 1942). This system is discussed in Chapter 15.

CLINICAL PICTURE

The metastasis may be silent for a long period. More often, pain and tenderness are prominent symptoms. Pathological fracture is fairly common.

Widespread bone destruction leads to an increase in serum calcium and an excess urinary excretion of calcium. Renal deposition is not uncommon. When renal damage is severe, leading to retention of phosphate, the serum phosphorus level may be raised. In the presence of widespread osteoblastic reaction and/or pathological fractures, serum alkaline phosphatase is often high.

RADIOGRAPHIC PICTURE

Secondary deposits are usually multiple. When they are solitary, problems of differential diagnosis may be insoluble by radiography. The lesions are generally small and they do not tend to spread much beyond the bone, so that large extra-osseous masses are not formed. There are, however, exceptions to these generalizations.

The reaction between cancer cells and host bone may be osteolytic, osteoblastic, and/or expansion of host bone. These features may be present singly or in different combinations in the same case. None of them necessarily occurs immediately or within any definite time limit after bone invasion. In fact, widespread infiltration into the interstices of spongy bone may be present for an appreciable period before there is radiographically visible alteration of normal bone pattern.

Osteolytic Changes

These show as irregular areas of bone destruction with edges that may present sharp definition or unmarginated fuzziness. Many small zones, appearing like punched-out holes of different sizes, may disturb cortical and calvarial shadows and remain discrete before ultimate fusion. Kidney, thyroid, and many breast carcinomata commonly produce osteolytic metastases.

Osteoblastic Changes

Osteoblastic changes involving endosteal as well as periosteal tissue may be demonstrated by radiography. Endosteal sclerosis is rather more common than are periosteal reactions, which may produce Codman's triangles and spiculation. The latter occasionally shows a rough, radiating sun-ray pattern. More exceptional still is a laminated form. Prostatic and bronchogenic cancers tend to produce osteoblastic lesions. Breast tumours are not uncommonly in this class.

Cortical Expansion

Bulging is uncommon. When it does occur, it tends to be slight or moderate in extent.

DIFFERENTIAL DIAGNOSIS

The differentiation from primary bone tumours may present difficulties, especially when the metastasis is solitary. Some of the main points are tabulated in *Table XXXVI*, p. 109.

Table XXXVI.—Differential Diagnosis—Metastatic and
Primary Bone Tumour

	Metastatic	Primary
No. of lesions . .	Usually multiple	Often single
Size of lesion . .	Usually small	Often large
Extra-osseous extension .	Seldom marked	Usually marked
Site of lesion . .	Predilection is notable (*Fig.* 15)	Sites are largely different from metastatic
Osteoblastic response .	Mainly endosteal	Periosteal often prominent

Carcinoma of Breast

The importance of carcinoma of the breast as a common source of osseous metastases has been noted. The latent interval between radical surgical removal of the breast and the appearance of metastases varies from weeks to decades.

The rate of spread in bone is often a reflection of the grade of malignancy of the primary. Equally often, the rate of progress, particularly during the earlier period, is hormone-dependent. Ovariectomy, adrenalectomy, or hypophysectomy usually has a marked effect on skeletal secondaries; partial healing occurs and may endure for an appreciable period, up to 3 years or so.

Osteolytic metastases are more common. They may occur alone or in association with osteoblastic reactions. Lytic lesions are more destructive than are sclerotic reactions, and surgical or medical inactivation of oestrogenic hormones often converts lytic into sclerotic responses.

Multiple foci are present in most cases of skeletal metastases from breast cancer. Geschickter (1945) found that about 1 in 4 was a solitary lesion. The vertebrae are probably most commonly affected, followed by the pelvis, ribs, 'upper' femora, skull, and 'upper' humeri, in that order.

Pain is the important clinical manifestation but it may be absent for a long time in proven foci. Vertebral secondaries may cause pain radiating along the peripheral distribution of a spinal nerve.

Two forms of treatment offer good, though temporary, alleviation of pain and bring about a transitory stay or recession of metastatic lesions. X-ray therapy has been used successfully for this purpose and alteration of the endocrine status can play a prominent role in management. Assessments of the value of administration of hormones differ to some extent in different centres. The A.M.A. Council's views (issued in 1951, and still widely applicable) may be summarized as follows:

Androgens

With testosterone propionate and methyl testosterone, used in both pre- and post-menopausal cases, there was some degree of subjective improvement in 80 per cent and objective improvement in 20 per cent. The mean duration of improvement was 1 year.

OESTROGENS

Generally, their use is confined to post-menopausal cases of at least 3 years' standing. Earlier use carries the danger of aggravating and increasing the extent of metastases. About 40 per cent showed some improvement and lived for an average of 15 months as compared with 8 months in those cases not so treated.

Appraisal of the effects of surgical or radiological ablation of endocrine organs also varies from centre to centre. The following indicates the average findings:—

OOPHORECTOMY

About one-third of patients show regression of metastases. An additional one-fifth have symptomatic improvement.

ADRENALECTOMY

In cases already helped by castration, but which show recrudescence and advance after a period of relief, adrenalectomy offers a further period of palliation in one-third to one-half. A small proportion of patients, not relieved by oophorectomy, is improved by adrenalectomy.

HYPOPHYSECTOMY

The results largely parallel those of castration.

Carcinoma of the Prostate

The special feature about skeletal spread is the tendency to the formation of osteoblastic lesions. Most frequently involved are the lumbar vertebrae and the pelvic bones; but other bones, like the skull and 'upper' femora, are also quite commonly invaded. An increase in serum acid phosphatase is usual but not invariable.

It is much more common in prostatic than in mammary cancer for bony metastases to provide the first indication of the presence of the disease. Low-back pain is a common herald.

Hormonal influence upon metastases is marked in about 90 per cent of cases and palliative therapy directed to the reduction or negation of androgenic influence is widely practised. The most popular form at present is castration combined with the exhibition of oestrogens. Adrenalectomy is a useful addition when the beneficial effects of the first two measures wear off.

Cancer of the Thyroid

Not infrequently the bone secondary is the presenting feature, and a pathological fracture may announce the condition.

The metastasis is osteolytic in character and, radiographically, usually presents as a well-defined translucency with or without loculation, and frequently with some expansion of the bone. The order of predilection of bones is skull, vertebrae, and pelvis. These three sites account for about two-thirds of the metastases. Other bones, like the femur, clavicle, sternum, ribs, etc., are also affected.

Papillary carcinoma of the thyroid is the type particularly prone to spread to osseous tissue. Many authors have remarked on the unique cytological change which not uncommonly occurs in osseous deposits, viz., the greater maturity, or differentiation, of the cancer cells by comparison with what is found in the primary.

A further peculiarity is the relative frequency of a solitary metastasis. This has led to surgical management by local removal of the bone lesion and thyroidectomy, with a reasonable though small chance of successful cure. X-ray therapy of bone lesions is of marked value; objective and subjective improvement may endure for a number of years.

Cancer of the Lung

The special tendency is the formation of multiple osteolytic lesions. Whereas the other ossophile cancers very rarely give rise to metastases in peripheral limb bones, bronchogenic cancers do so rather more often.

The prognosis is invariably very bad and palliation is seldom achieved.

Carcinoma of the Kidney

The skeletal metastases not infrequently proclaim the disease. The 'upper' femur is at the top of the list of frequency, followed by the other long bones, skull, vertebrae, and ribs. Solitary lesions may be amenable to surgical extirpation.

Radiologically, the lesion is translucent, indicating its osteolytic character. It is often extensive within bone and beyond it. The shadow may be generally cloudy or multiloculated.

Neuroblastoma

This tumour of early childhood has a special proclivity to metastasize to bones, particularly of the skull. Combined osteolytic and osteoblastic reactions are common. Erosions coexist with periosteal new bone formation. The latter is often of the radiating spicule pattern.

REFERENCES

ABRAMS, H. L., SPIRO, R., and GOLDSTEIN, N. (1950), 'Metastases in Carcinoma: Analysis of 1,000 Autopsied Cases', *Cancer*, **3**, 74.
A.M.A. COUNCIL OF PHARMACY AND CHEMISTRY (1951), 'Current Status of Hormone Therapy of Advanced Mammary Cancer', *J. Am. med. Ass.*, **146**, 47.
BATSON, O. V. (1940), 'The Function of Vertebral Veins and their Role in the Spread of Metastases', *Ann. Surg.*, **112**, 138.
— — (1942), 'The Role of the Vertebral Veins in Metastatic Processes', *Ann. intern. Med.*, **16**, 38.
COPELAND, M. M. (1931), 'Bone Metastases: Study of 334 Cases', *Radiology*, **16**, 198.
FORT, W. A. (1935), 'Cancer Metastatic to Bone', *Ibid.*, **24**, 96.
GESCHICKTER, C. F. (1945), *Diseases of the Breast*, 2nd ed. Philadelphia: Lippincott.
JAFFE, H. L. (1958), *Tumors and Tumorous Conditions of the Bones and Joints*. Philadelphia: Lea & Febiger.
McGRAW, J. P. (1965), 'Metastatic Lesions in Bone: General Discussion', in *Tumors of Bone and Soft Tissue*. Chicago: Year Book Medical Publishers.
WILLIS, R. A. (1941), 'A Review of 500 Consecutive Cancer Necropsies', *Med. J. Aust.*, **2**, 258.

CHAPTER 14

TUMOURS OF SYNOVIUM

SYNOVIAL CHONDROMATOSIS

THIS is a condition in which nodules and villi of cartilage form in the synovial membrane of a joint. Calcification and ossification may occur in some of the chondromata and this has led to an alternative name, viz., osteochondromatosis.

The condition is rare. It affects males more often, and mainly in the 20–40-year age-group. Most cases occur in a knee-joint. Occasionally it is bilateral and, in a small proportion of cases, large joints other than the knee are involved.

CLINICAL PICTURE

Pain and swelling are the initial clinical phenomena. Chondromatous bodies, either still attached or lying free, may cause locking of the joint, instability, clicks, and crepitations, and give rise to repeated episodes of acute traumatic synovitis.

Joint swelling is readily appreciable physically. It consists of synovial thickening, free fluid, and a general bogginess. Palpation during passive and active movement reveals the presence of multiple bodies of different sizes, resistance getting in the way of smooth gliding action, and crowding of the joint space.

RADIOGRAPHIC PICTURE

There is clouding of the joint cavity and, occasionally, small and faint opaque markings. Clear, multiple, rounded ossified bodies may be found with other loose bodies but are not part of the picture of chondromatosis.

MORBID ANATOMY

Nodules, pendent villi, and/or studs of cartilage, of different sizes and concentration project from a thickened synovial membrane. Some may become disconnected and lie free within the joint. On section, a number may show small areas of central calcification and/or ossification.

MORBID HISTOLOGY

Cartilage forms beneath the cells lining the synovial membrane. The chondroma grows actively and forms a nodule. If calcification and ossification occur, they begin within the centrum of a chondroma.

TREATMENT

Synovectomy with removal of chondromata is the treatment of choice.

SYNOVIAL HAEMANGIOMA

This rare tumour also affects the knee more often than it affects any other joint. The haemangioma is seldom confined to the synovium. It extends to periarticular structures, sometimes to the capsule and ligaments, and occasionally to bone.

Pain and limitation of movement are usual. Haemorrhage into the joint produces an acute attack of pain, swelling, and interference with function.

The haemangioma may be localized and encapsulated or it may lack definition and spread irregularly in the tissues. The vessels may be capillary or cavernous in type. The localized variety is amenable to complete excision but, for the diffuse lesion, only the more heavily involved areas can be removed.

Very occasionally, a tendon-sheath may be the seat of a haemangioma.

PIGMENTED VILLONODULAR SYNOVITIS

In 1941 Jaffe, Lichtenstein, and Sutro, suggested this name for a group of benign lesions affecting joints, bursae, tendon-sheaths, and juxta-tendinous structures. The 'synovitis' in the title indicates the authors' belief that the condition is essentially inflammatory. Other authorities (Willis, 1960) regard it as neoplastic and use the term 'benign synovioma'. The older titles 'xanthoma' and 'giant-cell tumours' are also still in use.

INCIDENCE

It is not uncommon.

SEX

Knee-joint lesions are more common in males. Tendon-sheath lesions are more common in females.

AGE

Most cases present in the age-group 20–50 years.

SITE

Localized lesions occur in the knee-joint (seldom in other joints), tendon-sheaths, and peritendinous structures, especially of the fingers, but also of the hands, the wrist, the feet, and the toes.

In a series of 118 cases, Jones, Soule, and Coventry (1969) found 91 in the fingers, 12 in the hand, wrist, and foot, 1 in the hip-joint, and 14 in the knee-joint. In the fingers, the most common location was adjacent to the distal interphalangeal joint.

Diffuse lesions affect the knee-joint, rarely tendon-sheaths and, in the occasional cases of bursal affection, diffuse lesions are the more common.

CLINICAL PICTURE

Pain and swelling are the main symptoms. They are mild for a long period, so that the condition has usually endured for some years before medical advice is sought. In the knee-joint, acute attacks with sharp pain and increased synovial effusion occur when adjacent joint surfaces nip villous tissue during weight-bearing movement.

In the series reported by Jones and others (1969) idiopathic or traumatic degenerative disease of joints features as a common associated pathology, and the question of an aetiological connexion stems from this association.

RADIOGRAPHIC PICTURE

A distended knee-joint and cloudy, cotton-wool, ball shadows are not uncommonly found. In the fingers, apart from evidence of degenerative arthritis, there may be signs of pressure decalcification in the neighbourhood of the tumour.

MORBID ANATOMY

In the earlier stages, synovial proliferations, of nodular and villous form, are distinct. Later the villi fuse or come to be crowded together to form a thick, matted, or spongy surface. The colour varies from reddish (where vascularity is rich) to brown (where there is haemosiderin) and to yellow (where there are lipid-containing cells).

MORBID HISTOLOGY

Synovial cells line the villi. Where villi are tangled and compressed together, cleft-like spaces lined by synovium are created. Within the lining, the stroma is rich in capillaries and the cells are plump, and ovoid or polyhedral in shape. Haemosiderin is found in these stroma cells, in the synovial lining cells, and also outside the cells. Lipid-containing cells are common, and they are often clumped together in foci of foam cells. Giant cells are frequent and they, too, may contain both haemosiderin and lipid. Strands of fibrosis are common within the villi. They may increase sufficiently to compress the usual rich cellular content into limited zones. Fibrosis may be preceded by the appearance of myxomatous areas. These may represent early collagen formation.

If the condition is neoplastic, its essential benignity is attested by the absence of metastases. If it is inflammatory, it is difficult to explain the rich cellularity, the increase in mitotic activity, the local invasive character sometimes exhibited, and the local recurrence after incomplete removal. Willis (1960) states that it may be both: an initial hyperplastic synovial reaction with subsequent neoplastic behaviour.

TREATMENT AND PROGNOSIS

Total extirpation of all synovium-bearing villi is called for. Anything less will be followed by recurrence. Localized lesions are usually amenable to complete removal, but diffuse involvement raises difficulties. Recurrences may be attacked surgically again, but it is noteworthy that X-ray therapy is often successful in controlling recurrences.

MALIGNANT SYNOVIOMA OR SYNOVIAL SARCOMA

This tumour probably arises from synovium, but tends to grow into peri-articular structures rather than into the joint. It has, in fact, been recorded in tissues at some distance away from a joint. Then it is supposed to arise from bursal synovial lining or from tissue with potential bursa-forming properties.

INCIDENCE

In a series of 449 cases of soft-tissue tumours, Martin, Butler, and Albores-Saavedra (1965) report 12 synovial sarcomata, i.e., rather less than 3 per cent.

Cade (1962) records a much higher incidence: 100 synovial sarcomata in a total of 366 soft-tissue sarcomata, i.e., about 26 per cent.

AGE

It occurs mainly during the third and fourth decades of life.

SEX

It is equally distributed.

SITE

The greatest number has been reported in the lower limb, the ratio relative to the upper limb being 3 : 1 or 4 : 1. The knee region heads the list, followed by the shoulder, hand, and foot, and then the elbow and other sites.

CLINICAL PICTURE

The early symptoms may be mild and thus ignored for a variable period from a few weeks to a few years. A painless swelling is usually the earliest sign. The swelling, when small and on the hand or foot, may be mistaken for a ganglion or a bursitis. When the swelling is large, it is soft and may give the sign of fluctuation. Tenderness is usually slight.

RADIOGRAPHIC PICTURE

The joint space is seldom involved and free fluid is not present. Bone invasion is also exceptional. When it occurs, it is osteolytic in type. Thus the radiographic picture, in the main, is one of an extra-articular shadow with an ill-defined outline and a general homogeneity of density except for opaque specks where calcification has taken place.

Neither the clinical nor the radiographic presentations offers much help in diagnosis, and the main prop in recognition is the histological picture.

MORBID ANATOMY

The gross characters vary considerably with localization and grade of malignancy. However, the false capsule created by compression of neighbouring tissues is fairly constant. The tumour mass tends to grow away from the joint and seldom encroaches on it. The consistency varies from that of soft jelly to firm rubber. It tends to grow irregularly by finger-like extensions into and between surrounding structures.

On cut section it is mainly grey-yellow in colour, but with reddish areas of haemorrhage, grey jelly-like mucinous zones, and irregular cystic spaces. Small foci of calcification are common.

MORBID HISTOLOGY

The two main components of synovial membrane, viz., the inner secretory pseudo-villous layer and the outer one of fibrous tissue, contribute in varying proportions to the cytological composition of the neoplasm. The picture may be predominantly fibrosarcomatous or pseudo-epithelial in different tumours or in different parts of one lesion.

The fibrosarcomatous element is basically composed of fusiform, spindle-shaped cells with collagen and reticulin fibres.

The secretory element presents several types of cells and several different arrangements. Many cells are plump and rounded, showing variations in size and shape; others are epithelial-like with cuboidal and columnar shapes. There may be areas where the cells have no particular arrangement but, characteristically, there are aggregations producing solid cords and apparent villi which project into clefts and irregular lacunae. The clefts come to be lined by the pseudo-epithelial cells which, in this situation, are often cuboidal or columnar, giving the impression of a glandular structure with acini and ductules. The cells lining clefts and spaces, whatever their shape, have no basement membrane, and the deeper cells have no recognizable organization. The pseudo-epithelial cells secrete a mucoid substance which is found within the clefts.

SPREAD

The rate of direct extension varies with the type and grade of malignancy. Disturbance of the pseudo-capsule, as by partial removal, biopsy, etc., may release a relatively controlled tumour and initiate a florid extension.

Lymphatic spread to regional nodes is fairly common, occurring in about 1 in 5 cases (Ariel and Pack, 1963). Even more frequent is haematogenous metastasization, particularly to the lungs. Here there may be discrete, cannon-ball lesions or wide infiltration. Other viscera and bones are also involved by blood-borne metastases.

DIFFERENTIAL DIAGNOSIS

Many difficult problems enter the diagnostic field and, not infrequently, detract from the possibility of early curative treatment.

A synovioma in the hand, wrist, or foot presents an obvious swelling at an early stage. Clinically it may be confused with a number of benign conditions, particularly a ganglion or giant-cell tumour of a tendon-sheath. Even at surgical exploration the presence of an apparently complete capsule may compound the confusion. The cytological composition, studied at a number of sites of the tumour, provides the answer.

A synovioma, remote from a joint, may be mistaken for a benign tumour (e.g., lipoma and mixed-tissue tumours designated fibrolipoma or fibromyxolipoma) and also for a malignant neoplasm (e.g., fibrosarcoma). Again, adequate histological examination is necessary for differentiation.

In the region of large joints, and especially the knee, bursitis and inflammatory lesions are among the non-neoplastic conditions to be considered. The benign pigmented villonodular synovitis presents confusing features. The points of distinction are outlined in *Table XXXVII*, p. 117.

TREATMENT AND PROGNOSIS

The prognosis is generally poor because of the frequency of metastases and the fact that they are often present by the time the relatively symptom-free condition appears for treatment. Cade (1962) records one of the most successful 'survival' rates in a large series. In 100 cases there was survival for 5 years or more in 56 and, of this number, 28 were free of recurrence. Ariel and Pack (1963) report a 29 per cent 5-year survival rate in a series of 25 patients.

When the tumour has remained localized and there are no metastases, radical, wide excision is called for. Neighbouring and adjacent structures, like muscles and tendons, are removed with the tumour mass. If removal of this extent of tissue jeopardizes the limb or severely limits its function, it is preferable to amputate well above the tumour level.

In the presence of lymph-node involvement, radical local block excision and/or amputation are still of value.

Table XXXVII.—DIFFERENTIAL DIAGNOSIS—SYNOVIOMA AND PIGMENTED VILLONODULAR SYNOVITIS

	SYNOVIOMA	VILLONODULAR SYNOVITIS
Pain . .	Pain mild or absent. No acute attacks	Mild pain with acute attacks
Intra-articular effusion	Absent	Often present
Radiography .	Shadow mainly extra-articular Specks of calcification	Usually intra-articular No calcification
Cytology .	Two components—fibrosarcoma and pseudo-epithelial	Many cells with haemosiderin and/or lipid. Giant cells present
Clefts . .	'Papillary' intrusions lined by epithelioid cells	Appear with compression and fusion; lined by small flat cells

Radiotherapy is a valuable adjunct to surgery. Some use it preoperatively as well as postoperatively, and it may be used together with, or as an alternative to, lymph-node excision. It is also used to palliate pulmonary and other haematogenous metastases.

Chemotherapy is still under investigation. Nitrogen mustard preparations and actinomycin D have been used. Claims for their value as part of a combined treatment have not yet been established.

REFERENCES

ARIEL, I. M., and PACK, G. T. (1963), 'Synovial Sarcoma', *New Engl. J. Med.*, **268**, 1272.

CADE, S. (1962), 'Synovial Sarcoma', *J. R. Coll. Surg. Edinb.*, **8**, 1.

JAFFE, H. L., LICHTENSTEIN, L., and SUTRO, C. J. (1941), 'Pigmented Villonodular Synovitis, Bursitis and Tenosynovitis', *Archs Path.*, **31**, 731.

JONES, F. E., SOULE, E. H., and COVENTRY, M. B. (1969), 'Fibrous Xanthoma of Synovium (Giant-Cell Tumor of Tendon Sheath, Pigmented Nodular Synovitis)', *J. Bone Jt Surg.*, **51A**, 76.

MARTIN, R. G., BUTLER, J. J., and ALBORES-SAAVEDRA, J. (1965), 'Soft Tissue Tumors: Surgical Treatment and Results', in *Tumors of Bone and Soft Tissue*. Chicago: Year Book Medical Publishers.

WILLIS, R. A. (1960), *Pathology of Tumours*, 3rd ed. London: Butterworths.

CHAPTER 15

TUMOURS OF THE VERTEBRAL COLUMN

BOTH primary and secondary neoplasms affect the vertebral column. Metastatic carcinoma is the commonest, both as an apparently isolated solitary tumour as well as an obvious multiple affection (Arseni, Simionescu, and Horwath, 1959; Cohen, Dahlin, and MacCarty, 1964). Multiple metastatic lesions are much more common than single metastases. Lodwick (1965) finds that more than 75 per cent of metastatic growths are multiple.

The great majority of all vertebral skeletal tumours are malignant in a proportion of about 4 or 5 : 1 as compared with those that are benign. This figure is all the more remarkable when it is recalled that the vertebral column is more commonly affected by metastases than any other bony site (Copeland, 1931; Fort, 1935).

METASTATIC CARCINOMA

INCIDENCE AND ORIGIN

The relative frequency of primary sites from which neoplasms spread to the vertebral column is variously reported. Delclos (1965) records the main three sites as breast 35 per cent, prostate 13 per cent, and lung as 12 per cent. The sites contributing the remaining percentages are head and neck, skin and lip, gastro-intestinal tract, cervix, kidney and bladder, thyroid, and miscellaneous and unknown. Lodwick's estimate differs somewhat in according the prostate a greater danger of 30 per cent. He suggests, too, that parallel with the increase in incidence of lung cancer, vertebral metastases from it will show progressively increasing proportions.

Abrams (1950) and other workers (Young and Funk, 1953) have found high rates of skeletal metastases in advanced cases. These include a large proportion of vertebral localizations. Necropsy examinations showed bony involvement in 84 per cent of deaths from prostatic carcinoma and in 73 per cent of females dying from breast cancer.

MODE OF SPREAD

The frequency of vertebral involvement and the high proportion this site contributes to the overall total of skeletal secondary growths are explicable on an anatomical basis.

In the first place, the route of spread is via the blood-stream. There is no evidence for any of the other forms of spread, either by direct continuity or by lymphatic channels. The question of which system of blood-vessels conveys the malignant cells points to the venous side. Vertebral metastases often occur in the absence of secondaries in other sites richly fed by the systemic arterial circulation. The lungs have a special relevance in this reasoning, because if tumour cells spread via arteries, the lungs would exhibit early and extensive evidence of seeding out; whereas, in fact, it often follows only some time after vertebral implantation.

Furthermore, other systemic arterial sites, such as other bones and soft structures, might be expected to show a rate of secondary involvement approaching that of the vertebrae, but, in fact, they do not.

Batson (1940, 1942) demonstrated the significance of a special system of veins related to the axial part of the skeleton, namely the vertebral column, the skull, and the pelvis. This has been called the vertebral system of veins. It has extensive and free intercommunications with the caval system, and flow between the two systems is constantly and physiologically subject to reversal of direction.

Veins are arranged in a segmental pattern in the vertebral column. At each vertebral level there are epidural and perivertebral plexuses collecting tributaries from bone, spinal cord, and other soft tissues, and then joining together to form intervertebral veins. At each intervertebral space, these latter veins communicate with segmental veins of the thoraco-abdominal wall, with the caval system, and with veins of the pelvis and the head and neck. Connexions also occur with pulmonary and azygos veins, and occasionally with portal and renal veins. Longitudinal veins connect the transversely disposed veins at vertebral segmental levels, so establishing a free system from the skull to the coccyx.

At the base of the skull, the vertebral system has free communications with the great dural sinuses which ultimately drain the brain, meninges, and diploë of the skull. By such channels, further connexions exist with emissary veins and extracranial veins and plexuses. Most of the veins of the skull, head, and neck drain into the internal jugulars, thus creating a great lake of venous blood in which flow currents are readily reversible.

At the caudal end of the vertebral system, an extensive plexus of veins lies on the anterior surfaces of the sacrum and coccyx, the lumbar vertebrae, and the iliac bones. The plexus receives tributaries from the neighbouring bones and has numerous communications with veins of the pelvic viscera. Batson reported that injection in the cadaver of the dorsal vein of the penis, a vein which freely inosculates with prostatic and retropubic plexuses, brought early filling of the pelvic sacrococcygeal plexuses.

The pelvic system is freely linked via the longitudinal vertebral veins with the vertebral system higher up; and, together with the rich anastomoses it has with the caval system, the great lake of venous blood is extended from head and neck down the vertebral system to the caudal reaches of the trunk.

Relative filling and emptying and changes in the direction of flow in these vast intercommunicating caval and vertebral venous complexes are subject to physiological and pathological influences. The negative intrathoracic pressure of every act of inspiration increases flow from the great caval veins into the heart, and thereby induces relative emptying of the vertebral system; consideration of the alternation of expiration with its increased intrathoracic pressure and therefore outflow from intrathoracic veins into the vertebral system makes the constancy of the to-and-fro current of venous blood between caval and vertebral systems very obvious. The direction of movement of blood is not the same at all levels of the trunk at any one time. Deep inspiration diminishes intrathoracic pressure and thereby activates flow from vertebral system into thoracic caval veins; but there is a synchronous increase in intra-abdominal pressure, giving rise to venous flow from the abdominal caval system into the lumbar and pelvic areas of the vertebral system. Changes of posture, some forms of exercise, and normal grades of abdominal strain will all influence the direction of flow of venous blood. It is also readily appreciable that pathological obstructions, particularly to the caval veins, affect the course taken by venous blood.

Malignant cells that have gained direct entry into a tributary of the vertebral system, as well as neoplastic emboli that have invaded the caval system and have been shunted into vertebral veins, may seed themselves in any of the bones of the axial skeleton.

CLINICAL PICTURE

Pain is the outstanding symptom. It is common locally and is also often referred to the distribution of a peripheral nerve. Tenderness is a frequent accompaniment. Paralyses and sensory changes result from nerve-root involvement.

RADIOGRAPHIC PICTURE

More often than not, multiple foci of spread are evident, making the diagnosis of metastatic disease probable. However, there are two circumstances in which recognition may be difficult. Firstly, widespread secondaries in the vertebral bodies may not show on radiography because of the absence of bone destruction or bone formation. Secondly, a solitary lesion, either apparent or real, is not uncommon; a circumstance which raises problems of differentiation from a primary bone tumour.

Metastases in the vertebrae tend to be small and remain within the medullary cavity. Soft-tissue extension is thus uncommon. The main characters differentiating metastases from primary neoplasms are indicated in *Table XXXVI*, p. 109. Differentiation from osteomyelitis is aided by its common extension to the disk, whereas, in malignant tumours, the disk is almost invariably spared.

The treatment of vertebral secondaries does not differ essentially from that for general skeletal affection, and this is discussed in Chapter 13.

NON-CARCINOMATOUS TUMOURS
CHORDOMA

This is one of the commonest of the primary malignant tumours of the vertebral column. It is described in Chapter 12.

MYELOMA

Cohen, Svien, and Dahlin (1964) present a series of 55 cases of myeloma of the vertebrae. About 60 per cent were situated in the thoracic region, 20 per cent in the lumbar, and the remainder in the cervical and sacral segments.

The two major forms of treatment used were ionizing radiation for pain and surgical decompression for paraplegia. A remarkable feature was the long survival time, 5–21 years, in 18 of the patients.

The modern attitude to the place of radiotherapy *vis-à-vis* chemotherapy in the management of myeloma is outlined in Chapter 11.

CHONDROSARCOMA

The occurrence is uncommon as it contributes less than 5 per cent of tumours of the vertebral column, and it is an unusual location for such tumours (*see* Chapter 5).

Pain and neurological disturbances are the common clinical features, and radiological examination often suggests a positive diagnosis. The pathological characters are no different in a vertebra than in other bones.

Complete ablation is the treatment of election at other sites, but it is difficult to achieve in a vertebral site. The prognosis is consequently worse than it is elsewhere.

GIANT-CELL TUMOUR

This still more uncommon primary neoplasm of the vertebrae has, in this region, a predilection for the sacrum.

Clinical, pathological, and other aspects of the neoplasm are the same as at its other locations and are detailed in Chapter 9.

BENIGN OSTEOBLASTOMA

The tumour is an uncommon one, but it has its highest incidence in the vertebral column. Here it gives rise to local pain and neurological disturbances. The diagnosis may be suggested by radiological examination, which demonstrates quite considerable expansion of the involved bone, and the translucency interrupted in places by calcification. Treatment is by excision of as much tumour as is practicable followed by irradiation.

ANEURYSMAL BONE CYST

This is also generally an uncommon tumour of bone, but 25–30 per cent of these cysts occur in the vertebral column. It has a good prognosis following surgical eradication of as much tumour as permitted by its situation.

EWING'S AND OTHER SARCOMA

Ewing's tumour is rare. Cytological study is necessary for diagnosis. Its treatment is largely palliative. Equally rare are *lymphomata* of all types, and their prognosis is also very poor. *Osteogenic sarcoma* contributes about 1 per cent of vertebral tumours. So, too, does *fibrosarcoma*. Other types of sarcoma, e.g., angiosarcoma, are exceptional.

HAEMANGIOMA

According to some authors (Ghormley and Adson, 1941), haemangioma is a common finding in vertebrae on autopsy examination. But others (Jaffe, 1958) believe that these findings represent focal varicosities but that they are not true neoplasms. When they do occur as acceptable neoplasms or hamartomata, pain and neurological disturbances are common sequels. Irradiation is the treatment of choice. Surgical excision is sometimes called for.

The prognosis is good in so far as there is a very small mortality-rate from complications, but it is poor in as far as symptoms, especially back pain, are concerned.

Certain benign tumours, such as osteoid-osteoma, chondroma, fibrous dysplasia, and neurilemmoma, occur but rarely in the vertebral column. They require histological examination of representative specimens for diagnosis.

EPENDYMOMA

Arising from cord elements, ependymoma may occasionally invade the adjacent vertebral bone by direct extension. Clinically and radiologically the condition resembles a primary tumour of bone, and it requires exploration and microscopy to establish the true diagnosis.

REFERENCES

ABRAMS, H. L. (1950), 'Skeletal Metastases in Carcinoma', *Radiology*, **55**, 534.

ARSENI, C. N., SIMIONESCU, M. D., and HORWATH, L. (1959), 'Tumours of the Spine', *Acta psychiat. scand.*, **34**, 398.

BATSON, O. V. (1940), 'The Functions of Vertebral Veins and their Role in the Spread of Metastases', *Ann. Surg.*, **112**, 138.

— — (1942), 'The Role of the Vertebral Veins in Metastatic Processes', *Ann. intern. Med.*, **16**, 38.

COHEN, D. M., DAHLIN, D. C., and MacCARTY, C. S. (1964), 'Apparently Solitary Tumors of the Vertebral Column', *Proc. Staff Meet. Mayo Clin.*, **39**, 509.

— — SVIEN, H. J., and DAHLIN, D. C. (1964), 'Long Term Survival of Patients with Myeloma of the Vertebral Column', *J. Am. med. Ass.*, **187**, 914.

COPELAND, M. M. (1931), 'Bone Metastases: Study of 334 Cases', *Radiology*, **16**, 198.

DELCLOS, L. (1965), 'The Place of Radiotherapy in the Palliative Treatment for Bone Metastases', in *Tumors of Bone and Soft Tissue*. Chicago: Year Book Medical Publishers.

FORT, W. A. (1935), 'Cancer Metastatic to Bone', *Radiology*, **24**, 96.

GHORMLEY, R. K., and ADSON, A. W. (1941), 'Hemangioma of Vertebrae', *J. Bone Jt Surg.*, **39**, 887.

JAFFE, H. L. (1958), *Tumors and Tumorous Conditions of the Bones and Joints*. Philadelphia: Lea & Febiger.

LODWICK, G. S. (1965), 'The Radiological Diagnosis of Metastatic Cancer in Bone', in *Tumors of Bone and Soft Tissue*. Chicago: Year Book Medical Publishers.

YOUNG, J. M., and FUNK, F. J., jun. (1953), 'Incidence of Tumor Metastases to the Lumbar Spine: A Comparative Study of Roentgenographic Changes and Gross Lesions', *J. Bone Jt Surg.*, **35A**, 55.

CHAPTER 16

TUMOURS OF THE ODONTOGENIC APPARATUS AND JAWS

THESE tumours are a special group, pathologically and clinically. Many of them are peculiar to the jaws; some are but particular anatomical localizations of neoplasms that more commonly attack other bones; and not a few of the latter group have somewhat different effects and results when they occur in the jaws as compared with the rest of the skeleton.

In framing a classification three cardinal aspects exercise a deciding influence. The benign or malignant behaviour, the origin from odontogenic or other tissue, and the general composition in terms of cystic or solid forms are the three chief qualities leading to the following classification:—

1. *Benign odontogenic cysts.—*
   a. Radicular.
   b. Follicular.

2. *Benign non-odontogenic vestigial cysts.—*
   a. Median fissural cysts of the maxilla.
   b. Globulomaxillary.
   c. Nasopalatine.

3. *Benign non-odontogenic simple cysts.—*
   a. Solitary bone cyst.
   b. Aneurysmal bone cyst.

4. *Benign odontogenic tumours.—*
   a. Ameloblastoma (simple).
       i. Adeno-ameloblastoma.
       ii. Melano-ameloblastoma.
   b. Myxoma.
   c. Fibroma.
   d. Dentinoma.
   e. Cementoma.
   f. Cementifying fibroma.
   g. Ameloblastic fibroma and other mixed tumours.
   h. Odontoma.

5. *Benign non-odontogenic tumours.—*
   a. Torus.
   b. Osteoid osteoma.
   c. Fibrous dysplasia.
   d. Giant-cell reparative granuloma.
   e. Giant-cell tumour.

6. *Malignant tumours.*—
   a. Primary.
   b. Metastatic.

BENIGN ODONTOGENIC CYSTS
Radicular Cysts

These are also known as apical, dental, and periodontal cysts, and are the commonest cysts of the odontogenic apparatus, accounting for almost two-thirds of all cases (Fickling, 1965).

ORIGIN AND DEVELOPMENT

The first stage is an infection of the dental pulp which forms a dental or apical granuloma, in which epithelial remnants are caught up and enclosed. The clumps of epithelial debris become activated and proliferate, so removing part or all of the granuloma and converting it into a cyst lined by the epithelium. The cyst may enlarge from a diameter of 5 mm. or so to 10 cm. and involve a considerable mass of maxilla or mandible.

SITE

The upper jaw is affected more often than the lower, and the cyst may arise in deciduous, transitional, or permanent teeth. The granuloma and consequent cyst may be apical or lateral (periodontal) in location, and it may persist even after dental extraction.

CLINICAL PICTURE

Pain is the outstanding symptom and, since the condition has an inflammatory basis, persistent pain after removal of the affected tooth indicates a residual radicular cyst. The affected tooth and alveolus are tender and the area is often swollen.

RADIOGRAPHIC PICTURE

The clear translucent area about and beyond the apex of the tooth, or, less often, to one or both sides of it, is the constant finding. The outline of the cyst may be irregular with fuzzy extensions into adjacent bone or, in long-standing cases, it will resemble a chronic osteomyelitis and exhibit a smooth, sclerotic border. The tooth shows signs of caries and pulp infection, varying in extent with the duration of the condition.

MORBID HISTOLOGY

The cyst lining is squamous epithelium, which may show irregular proliferation. Although malignant change to squamous-cell epithelioma does not occur in this condition, the histological appearances may closely resemble such a tumour. Underlying the epithelium and for an appreciable depth, there is dense chronic inflammatory fibrosis.

Active inflammation is usual and shows by lymphocytic and plasma-cell infiltration of the cyst wall. Foreign-body giant cells are common and small sequestra may be found.

TREATMENT

The cyst wall should be completely removed to prevent recurrence or persistence.

Follicular Cysts

These are also known as dentigerous, multilocular, odontogenic, epithelial, and primordial cysts, and arise from abnormalities of dental development. Several types have been separately named.

The central follicular (dentigerous) cyst is the most common type. Most occur at the cuspid and third molar teeth; the incidence at this site being correlated with the frequency of abnormalities of eruption in these teeth.

The simple follicular or primordial cyst results from an encystment of fluid between the enamel layers of a tooth follicle. Here, too, disturbances of development, as by impaction of an unerupted tooth, may be the essential aetiological factor; but superimposed infection interfering with proper development may be an important agent.

The lateral follicular or periodontal cyst is uncommon. It arises by much the same mechanisms as the others, but its situation on the lateral aspect of the tooth gives it this name. The term 'periodontal' is used occasionally in the literature, but it should be abandoned here and reserved for the much more common periodontal radicular cyst.

The multilocular follicular cyst is rare. It arises from multiple epithelial rests of dentigerous origin. The rests enlarge and coalesce irregularly to produce this type of cyst.

INCIDENCE

In Fickling's (1965) series, follicular cysts, as here defined, accounted for about 25 per cent of all cysts of the jaws.

AGE

It may present in children, when it is assumed to have originated from odontogenic epithelium prior to the formation of enamel because there is no tooth crown associated with the cyst. In adults, when a crown is present, it points to the origin of the cyst at a later stage of dental development.

CLINICAL PICTURE

The cyst is often symptomless for a long period and may be discovered on radiography done for other reasons. Swelling and deformity occur late and dull pain may be the heralding feature. Infection may supervene and add its own clinical evidence.

RADIOGRAPHIC PICTURE

This is often diagnostic, demonstrating a well-defined, translucent cyst with a regular thin sclerotic surround. Spongy bone is first compressed and then cortex is thinned and expanded. In the adult type, the tooth is evident; in the young type, there is no tooth. The occasional multilocular cyst may be somewhat more difficult to differentiate from other conditions.

Morbid Anatomy and Histology

In the adult type, proper eruption of the affected tooth does not occur. In childhood the cyst is devoid of a tooth unless the cyst originated from an abnormal supernumerary dental element.

Squamous epithelium lines the lumen, and collagen or poorly organized fibrous tissue underlies the epithelium. Inflammatory changes may distort the cellular pattern. The fluid content may be clear or dark in colour, or it may be infected and purulent.

Odontogenic epithelial remnants are present in a high proportion, and this carries a risk of transformation (Bernier, 1960) to ameloblastoma (adamantinoma). The risk of tumorous change has also been reported by other authors (Sonesson, 1950; Bradfield and Broadway, 1958).

Treatment

Complete removal of all the cyst lining is curative and necessary to prevent recurrence and to remove the potential of transformation to other more dangerous tumours.

Benign Non-odontogenic Vestigial Cysts

These uncommon cysts occur at the sites and lines of fusion of the developing upper or lower jaw bones. The nomenclature applied is descriptive of the developmental zone affected.

Median Fissural Cysts of the Maxilla

An alternative name of midline palatal cyst is indicative of its position and the site of origin along the line of fusion of the palatal processes of the maxilla. It is more often located towards the anterior end of this line, presenting just behind the upper incisor teeth, and is there known as a median alveolar cyst.

Midline cysts of the mandible are more uncommon than those of the maxilla. They also usually present on the buccal aspect of the bone. The cyst arises from entrapped epithelial debris and grows to an average size of 1–3 cm. in diameter. Radiologically, a defect along the midline suture is usual, and, microscopically, the epithelium, stratified or bronchial, is the important component.

Globulomaxillary Cyst

The fusion line concerned is between the globular process or premaxilla of the frontonasal bone and the maxilla.

The cyst is originally removed from dental roots, but as it grows it encroaches on them. The teeth involved are the cuspid and the lateral incisor, which are separated and malalined by the cyst.

The swelling may present in the floor of the nose or into the alveolus, or in both directions. Radiography demonstrates its location which, as mentioned, bears a constant relationship to the teeth. Histological study reveals an epithelial lining which is often of a modified respiratory type, resembling that in the lining of the nose.

Nasopalatine Cysts

The cysts originate from epithelial remnants of the nasopalatine ducts and are of two varieties: the cyst of the incisive canal which presents high up in the maxillary process, and the cyst of the palatine papilla presenting at the oral opening of the nasopalatine canal. Radiologically, they are close to the midline and tend to assume a heart-shape, the apex being between the central incisors, and the indentation in the base being caused by the nasal spinous process.

Histological examination demonstrates an epithelial lining, either modified respiratory in type or squamous, or both. The presence of mucous glands in the cyst wall strongly favours a diagnosis of a nasopalatine cyst.

BENIGN NON-ODONTOGENIC SIMPLE CYSTS

Solitary Bone Cyst

A solitary cyst, similar to that found in long bones, and discussed in Chapter 3, very occasionally occurs in the jaws. As in other locations, so too in the jaws, it affects mainly the young.

Whilst trauma as an aetiological agent when the cyst arises in long bones has very little to sustain it, in the jaws there may be a more acceptable thesis that trauma is a factor of some weight. However, proof is difficult to establish.

Clinically, the bone is expanded and is often painful and tender. Pathological fractures of the thin walls of the cyst may bring it to first notice. Radiography shows an irregularly outlined cyst taking the general shape of the jaw bone affected and including the roots of the related teeth. The roots look like prongs dipping down into an empty cavity.

The cyst may be empty or contain clear to yellow or bloody fluid. Its wall is composed of thinned and expanded cortical bone and it is devoid of a lining membrane. Microscopically a fibrous tissue lining is usual, and there may be evidence of reactive bone formation.

Aneurysmal Bone Cyst

As elsewhere in the skeleton, aneurysmal bone cysts of the jaws occur, in the main, during the second decade of life.

Its pathology is similar to that described in the general discussion of the condition in Chapter 3. So, too, is the clinical picture except that, in the jaws, antecedent trauma, particularly dental extraction, is a common feature.

SURGICAL TECHNIQUES IN THE TREATMENT OF CYSTS

There are a number of different technical procedures used in dealing with cysts of the jaws.

1. Via an intra-oral incision, the cyst lining is completely removed. If it is certain that removal has been complete, and there is no infection, the wound may be closed. Otherwise, the cavity is packed.

2. In elderly patients or those suffering from some general condition which may interfere with healing, and when part of the cyst wall closely abuts against the maxillary sinus, the floor of the nose, the teeth, or the mandibular nerve, the cyst 'roof' or 'floor', i.e., its oral wall away from the structures to be guarded, is

completely removed. The remaining cyst cavity thus widely exposed is then lightly packed.

3. For the same indications, but when it is not possible to remove a wide area of one wall, a relatively small opening may be made and a plug inserted through it. This procedure is also useful as a first stage for a later complete enucleation.

4. For cysts presenting and possibly leaking into the maxillary sinus or the floor of the nose, the wide opening may be made in the sinus and nose.

5. Occasionally, when conditions of position and presentation of the cyst are appropriate, approach to it may be via a submandibular incision.

BENIGN ODONTOGENIC TUMOURS

Simple Ameloblastoma

This is also known as adamantinoma, epithelial odontoma, and soft odontoma. Since 'adamantinoma' implies the formation of enamel, which in fact is not present in the tumour, 'ameloblastoma' is becoming the preferred term.

The tumour arises from proliferation of ectodermal cells of the odontogenic apparatus, most probably from remnants of the dental lamina or outer enamel epithelium.

AGE

The peak period of incidence is from 20 to 35 years.

SEX

Males are more commonly affected than females.

SITE

It is nearly always situated in the mandible, and particularly at its angle, where some 75 per cent of these tumours occur (Bernier, 1960).

RACE INCIDENCE

Tumours of the jaws among native peoples of Central Africa are remarkably frequent. Burkitt's tumour accounts for a large proportion amounting to about 40 per cent, but, apart from this, other jaw tumours also have a high comparative incidence (Dodge, 1965). Ameloblastoma is particularly common as is clearly shown by the comparative tables produced by Anand, Davey, and Cohen (1967). In a number of regions of Africa, the frequency of ameloblastoma expressed as a percentage of all tumours in these regions varies from 0·6 to 2·7; compared to figures of 0·07 in whites and 0·15 in Negroes in the United States of America.

RELATION TO FOLLICULAR CYSTS

Bernier reports that 33 per cent of 88 cases of ameloblastoma arose in association with follicular cysts.

CLINICAL PICTURE

Slow painless growth is usual, leading to such gradual enlargement that the patient appreciates it only at an advanced stage. The mass often bulges to both inner and outer aspects, causing facial swelling and asymmetry, distortion of the dental arches, and displacement and loosening of the teeth. The surface remains smooth until the cortex is completely eroded, or there is recurrence after surgery.

Radiographic Picture

The area of translucency is clearly demarcated; it is often marked by the walls of multiple loculation. The cortex of adjacent bone is gradually expanded and thinned, and its density varies in different cases. The teeth are distorted and their roots are often 'shaved off'. With progression of the tumour, the clear outline becomes cloudy, and irregular calcific shadows occupy much of the mass. Finally, extensive bone destruction and loss of teeth become marked features.

Morbid Anatomy

The tumour may be large, up to several inches in diameter. For some years it appears encapsulated and has a roughly lobulated surface. Expansion of the bone is accompanied by compression and erosion of spongy and cortical bone. In advanced cases the cortex is destroyed so that the tumour comes to the surface. Infection is not infrequent in advanced cases, and sinuses, intra-oral or external on to the skin, may follow.

On cut section, the appearances vary from a solid granular surface to a multi-cystic one; sometimes both are present in one tumour.

Morbid Histology

Variation is also marked in the histological findings in different tumours and in different parts of one tumour. Ramifying and communicating cords of odontogenic cells are common. The margins of the cords or streams of cells stand out clearly by taking stain more deeply and by their cuboidal or columnar shape with basal nuclei. The cells may be tightly packed with areas of loosening in parts, giving a similar picture to that of the stellate reticulum of a tooth follicle. In the centre of a stream, the cells are generally polyhedral and, quite frequently, they liquefy and progress to form large cystic spaces.

The cells are set in a stroma varying from a loose arrangement of spindle-shaped connective-tissue cells to a more compact setting.

Not uncommonly, the odontogenic cells undergo metaplasia to a squamous type, and central keratinization is then a frequent by-product. When this is marked, the term 'acanthomatous ameloblastoma' may be used. The appearances may resemble those of a squamous-cell carcinoma, but it is very doubtful whether such malignant transformation ever occurs. The general consensus of opinion is that ameloblastoma is and remains a benign tumour.

Course

Quite commonly, recurrences follow surgical removal. This is a slow process and may take years to become manifest. It is almost certainly due to persistent growth of portions of the original tumour left behind at the operation.

Treatment

The frequency of local recurrence has led to more complete local resection at the first surgical attack. The tumour is completely removed with its capsule, with related periosteum, and with a margin of normal bone at both extremities. For large tumours, hemimandibulectomy or whole-jaw resection, with or without the condyles, is usually required.

Adeno-ameloblastoma

This is a rare tumour. It occurs mainly from 10 to 20 years and in the body of the mandible. As implied by the name, the cells are arranged in acinar and ductule patterns. There is no tendency to recur after local removal.

Melano-ameloblastoma

Melano-ameloblastoma arises during the first year of infancy and is almost invariably located in the frontal regions of the maxilla. Its cells contain melanin pigment. It may cause gross deformity, but it is benign and reacts well to local removal and curettage.

The question whether the tumour arises from retinal or dental elements is not yet resolved.

Myxoma

This benign odontogenic tumour of mesodermal origin usually begins in childhood or youth but grows so gradually and painlessly that it is commonly discovered later in life. It is often accompanied by displaced or missing teeth.

Histologically, the picture is of a small amount of connective-tissue fibres set in a granular mucoid matrix, with an admixture of scattered fibroblastic stellate cells that resemble primitive mesodermal tissue of the dental papilla.

It behaves in a benign manner and is amenable to local removal.

Fibroma

This is an odontogenic benign tumour differing but slightly from myxoma in that it has a richer fibrous tissue component, which is often arranged in strands and fascicles. The degree of cellularity varies, but it is questionable whether an odontogenic fibrosarcoma occurs. In certain African regions, these tumours may grow to grotesque sizes. Local excision is usually curative in the smaller lesions, but major resections may be necessary for the large ones.

Dentinoma

Whereas myxoma and fibroma originate from tissue of an early stage of odontogenesis, dentinoma arises at a later phase. Irregular calcification occurs in the maturing mesenchymal tissue, and dentine-like fibrillar structures become included in the matrix.

Cementoma

As with dentinoma, this takes origin at a late stage of odontogenesis. The tumour presents as a nodular aggregation of cementum, varying in size from a half to several centimetres, attached to the apex of a tooth. It is painless and remains hidden until an incidental radiological examination reveals it, or until it grows so large as to form an obvious lump.

Cementifying Fibroma

This is also a 'late' developer and is applied to cementum lying as unconnected accretions within a soft-tissue mass in the jaw bone. It is probably a form of fibrous dysplasia (*see* Chapter 4), and may be a variant of ossifying fibroma which also occurs in the jaws. The conditions are amenable to enucleation procedures.

Ameloblastic Fibroma

Ameloblastic fibroma is a mixed odontogenic tumour, arising from ectodermal and mesodermal elements. It is benign and slowly growing and, as with the other odontogenic tumours, it is usually found with missing or otherwise abnormally developed teeth.

This histological pattern characterizes the tumour, segregating it from simple ameloblastomata. Cords and islands of odontogenic epithelium, often well differentiated and sometimes arranged in masses resembling tooth buds, are associated with odontogenic connective tissue arranged, for the most part, in loose embryonic form like that of a dental papilla. Cyst formation is exceptional.

The prognosis following complete removal is good.

Ameloblastic Haemangioma and Neurilemmoma

Both are rare examples of mixed tumours. There is some doubt whether the haemangioma and neurilemmoma are of odontogenic origin or incidental accompanying elements of the ameloblastoma.

Ameloblastic Odontoma

This mixed tumour arises at a late phase of odontogenic development as evidenced by the presence of differentiation of the connective-tissue element to calcification, which forms cementum or dentine.

Odontoma

This fairly common, mixed, composite, odontogenic tumour often exhibits a grade of differentiation just short of full maturation.

The tumours are usually encapsulated and contain irregular masses of dentine, cementum, and enamel, with a suggestion of their organization, albeit irregular and primitive, towards a tooth.

The tumour is slow-growing and may reach massive proportions.

BENIGN NON-ODONTOGENIC TUMOURS

Exostosis

Exostosis, known in the jaws as torus maxillaris or torus mandibularis, is a common lesion, being found in about 20 per cent of the population (Bernier, 1960).

The maxilla, particularly close to the midline of the palate, bears most of them and the mandible a minority.

The exostosis consists of cortical bone with minimal stroma, and only in the large projections is there a medullary centrum.

Growth is absent or very slight. The lesions may require removal when they 'get in the way' or interfere with function.

Osteoid-osteoma

This occasionally affects the jaws; its characters, as described in Chapter 3, are the same as they are elsewhere in the skeletal system.

Fibrous Dysplasia

This is not common in the jaws, but the monostotic form is the type more often found. Notwithstanding the fact that in the jaws the condition bears similarities to that found in other bones (*see* Chapter 4), there are special manifestations of the disease which may be due to peculiarities of odontogenesis and the development of the jaws.

Although it arises before puberty, its slow progress usually delays discovery until later in life. Localized or massive parts of either maxilla or mandible may be affected. Pain arises late and deformity or enlargement heralds the condition.

The radiographic picture varies with the amount and distribution of fibrous and osseous components: the range is from small cystic areas with slight opacities to large irregular areas of opacity with little of the translucency of fibrous tissue zones. Confusion in diagnosis is frequent on a radiological basis and this is also not infrequently the case after histological examination. Representative segments of tissue from a number of different portions of the tumour require extensive study to reach a probable if not certain diagnosis.

The tumours lend themselves to 'shelling out', so that major procedures are seldom necessary.

Giant-cell Reparative Granuloma and Giant-cell Tumour

The two conditions belong to different classes of bone disease: the former is not neoplastic, but represents a focus of repair and healing; whereas the latter is a tumour occupying a pathological position on both sides of the border line between benign and malignant neoplasia. They are coupled here because of the importance of their differentiation from one another. There is a third condition, a metabolic endocrine effect of tumours of the parathyroid gland, which also presents as a bony tumefaction in the jaws and enters the present diagnostic field. The main features of differentiation are noted in *Table XXVII*, p. 79.

MALIGNANT TUMOURS OF THE JAWS

Sarcoma

Osteogenic sarcoma has been estimated to occur in 1 of every 75,000 persons in Great Britain (Platt, 1952) and 1 per 100,000 in the United States (Cade, 1952). Approximately 6·5 per cent of osteogenic sarcoma, together with fibroblastic and chondroblastic types, arise in the jaws (Garrington, Scofield, Corryn, and Hooker, 1967), giving a crude incidence in the United States of 0·07 per 100,000 population per year.

The general pathological, clinical, and diagnostic features of osteogenic sarcoma are reviewed in Chapter 6; fibrosarcoma and chondrosarcoma are dealt with in Chapters 7 and 5, respectively.

The special characters of the conditions as they present in the jaws concern their age and site incidence and prognosis. The peak age falls about a decade later than it does elsewhere in the skeleton, occurring in the jaws chiefly in the third decade.

An analysis of site in relation to age and sex, as found by Garrington and others, is of interest and possible significance. About two-thirds of their 56 cases had mandibular lesions and one-third maxillary. In the mandibular group, the age incidence was spread fairly evenly over the first five decades, with a minor peak during the second decade. In the maxilla, there was a sharp peak of tumour incidence during the third decade. There was a slight preponderance of males in the overall figures (31 : 24), but there were marked differences in relation to site. Of the 24 females, no less than 22 had lesions in the lower jaw, whereas there were roughly equal numbers of males suffering from upper and lower jaw lesions.

The location in the jaws (Garrington and others) is summarized in *Table XXXVIII.*

Table XXXVIII.—LOCATION OF BONE SARCOMA

Maxilla		Mandible	
Alveolus	8	Body and symphysis	27
Mid-anterior	4	Angle	6
Antrum	4	Vertical ramus	3

PROGNOSIS

The prognosis for the jaw affection is better than that for the tumour in other bones (Kragh, Dahlin, and Erich, 1958; Friedberg, Serlin, and Travaglini, 1962; Schwartz and Alpert, 1963). This is probably correlated with earlier recognition, with accessibility of the tumour, and the possibility for radical resection. The correlations are strengthened by the more favourable outlook for mandibular growths, which are more frequent, and the fact that the unusual antral lesions have the poorest prognosis in the group.

Ewing's Sarcoma

This tumour is discussed in Chapter 10. It is very uncommon in the jaws, and its characters here resemble those situated in other bones.

Myeloma

Occasionally, the solitary or multiple type may occur in the jaws, being located in the mandible less infrequently than in the maxilla. The manifestations and behaviour of myeloma in the jaw are similar to its occurrence elsewhere. The subject is discussed in Chapter 11.

Metastatic Tumours of the Jaws

Although metastases to the jaws are not common, there are records of such spread from carcinomata, sarcomata, and other tumours. The possibility has to be taken into account in assessing the differential diagnosis.

Burkitt's Tumour

The characters and manifestations of this lymphosarcomatous tumour were co-ordinated into a unified clinical entity by Burkitt (1958, 1962, 1963). It is probably a multicentric tumour, but lesions in the jaw bones are the commonest heralds of the disease, appearing in this site in 50–60 per cent of cases. Both the mandible and the maxilla are vulnerable; two quadrants are involved in more than half the cases, and all four quadrants in about 11 per cent. One of every three maxillary lesions extends to and distorts the orbit. Other situations, both osseous and extra-osseous, are frequently involved: abdominal nodes and viscera, almost invariably; the thyroid, testis, spine, and long bones, quite commonly.

The geographical distribution is peculiar; it has a high incidence in Central Africa. In Uganda, it constitutes more than half the malignant tumours of children; in Nigeria (Edington and Maclean, 1964), it is second only to cancer of the cervix in terms of all malignant disease diagnosed in Ibadan. In this same geographical area, Anand and others (1967) record that Burkitt's tumour contributed 102 out of a total of 135 cases of malignant tumours of bony and soft tissues of the jaws.

REFERENCES

ANAND, S. V., DAVEY, W. W., and COHEN, B. (1967), 'Tumours of the Jaw in West Africa', *Br. J. Surg.*, **54**, 901.

BERNIER, J. L. (1960), *Tumors of the Odontogenic Apparatus and Jaws*. Washington: Armed Forces Inst. of Path.

BRADFIELD, W. J. D., and BROADWAY, E. S. (1958), 'Malignant Change in a Dentigerous Cyst', *Br. J. Surg.*, **45**, 657.

BURKITT, D. (1958), 'A Sarcoma involving the Jaws in African Children', *Ibid.*, **46**, 218.

— — (1962), 'A Lymphoma Syndrome in African Children', *Ann. R. Coll. Surg.*, **30**, 211.

— — (1963), in *Cancer Progress Volume* (ed. RAVEN, R. W.). London: Butterworths.

CADE, S. (1952), *Malignant Disease and its Treatment by Radium*, 2nd ed. Baltimore: Williams & Wilkins.

DODGE, O. G. (1965), 'Tumours of the Jaw, Odontogenic Tissues and Maxillary Antrum (excluding Burkitt's Lymphoma) in Ugandan Africans', *Cancer*, **18**, 205.

EDINGTON, G. M., and MACLEAN, C. M. N. (1964), 'Incidence of the Burkitt Tumour in Ibadan, Western Nigeria', *Br. med. J.*, **1**, 264.

FICKLING, B. W. (1965), 'Cysts of the Jaw: A Long-term Survey of Types and Treatment', *Proc. R. Soc. Med.*, **58**, 847.

FRIEDBERG, M. J., SERLIN, O., and TRAVAGLINI, E. (1962), 'Osteosarcoma of the Maxilla', *Oral Surg.*, **15**, 883.

GARRINGTON, G. E., SCOFIELD, H. H., CORRYN, J., and HOOKER, S. P. (1967), 'Osteosarcoma of the Jaws', *Cancer*, **20**, 377.

KRAGH, L. V., DAHLIN, D. C., and ERICH, J. B. (1958), 'Osteogenic Sarcoma of the Jaws and Facial Bones', *Am. J. Surg.*, **96**, 496.

PLATT, H. (1952), 'Symposium on Sarcoma of Bone: Royal Society of Medicine', *J. Bone Jt Surg.*, **34B**, 322.

SCHWARTZ, D. T., and ALPERT, M. (1963), 'The Clinical Course of Mandibular Osteogenic Sarcoma', *Oral Surg.*, **16**, 769.

SONESSON, A. (1950), 'Odontogenic Cysts and Cystic Tumours of the Jaws', *Acta Radiol.*, Suppl. 81.

CHAPTER 17

TUMOURS OF THE HAND

TUMOURS of the hand may be divided into those affecting skeletal, joint, and extra-skeletal structures, but it is clinically appropriate to recall the close proximity and intimate association of soft and bony tissues.

SOFT-TISSUE TUMOURS

Ganglion

This, the commonest tumour of the hands, arises mainly about the wrist or over the flexor surface near the metacarpophalangeal joints. Carp and Stout (1928) discuss the many theories that have been propounded to explain its nature and origin; the issue is not yet finally decided. The basic pathology is probably a degeneration of fibrous tissue near a joint or tendon-sheath.

AGE

It presents mostly between the ages of 15 and 30 years.

SEX

More females are affected than males.

CAUSE

Trauma is probably a factor, especially minor, repeated, subclinical injury.

MORBID ANATOMY

The ganglion may consist of a single cyst or a collection of multiple small cysts. The clear, jelly-like content does not communicate with the adjacent joint or tendon-sheath synovial cavity. The non-specific lining of a ganglion is further evidence of its lack of connexion or origin from synovium. Malignant transformation has not been recorded.

CLINICAL PICTURE

The lump is the most obvious clinical feature. Pain and discomfort, when present, are not marked.

DIFFERENTIAL DIAGNOSIS

Aspiration of the typical content differentiates the ganglion from synovitis or tenosynovitis. On the dorsum of the distal interphalangeal joint, a mucous cyst or Heberden's node may be suspect; also other cysts and soft tumours may come into the picture, but they all lack the characteristic tenseness of the ganglion. Deeply situated lesions may have to await exploration and excision for final diagnosis.

TREATMENT

External rupturing force, various sclerosing injections, and a seton suture have been fashionable from time to time. Most ganglia recur after such treatment. They require adequate surgical exploration and complete excision in a bloodless field for successful cure.

Epidermoid Inclusion Cysts

In personal records, this comes next in the list of frequency of hand tumours. They are particularly common in industrial workers and among women machinists in clothing factories. It was the most frequent tumour seen in the hands of men employed at an abattoir; during a period of 15 years it outnumbered all other tumours by 3 to 1.

King (1933), among others, considers that the cysts are initiated by injury. A wound, incised, crushed, or penetrating, leads to implantation of epidermal cells, which then proliferate to produce a squamous-cell-lined cyst containing epithelial debris. The injury antedates the cyst by several months to a year or more. Occasionally they occur within the bony phalanx (Carroll, 1953a).

The cysts are cured by complete excision.

Xanthoma or Pigmented Villonodular Synovitis

These benign lesions affecting large joints, especially the knee and tendon-sheaths, are common in the wrist and fingers. The general characters, pathological and clinical, are noted in Chapter 14. The differential diagnosis from other tumours of the hands presents some problems on clinical appearances. Whilst it is firm, it does not possess the tense cystic fullness of a ganglion; other helpful features are its usual appearance some distance away from a joint, and its mobility in a lateral direction. A tightly encapsulated lipoma, gouty tophi, and chronic inflammatory masses may cause doubt, but operative exposure soon reveals the typical grey-yellow colour of the xanthoma together with the lines or aggregations of reddish-brown colour set in the tumour mass.

Phalen, McCormack, and Gazale (1959) found that in the hands it presented mainly in the fifth and sixth decades of life.

The treatment is local excision, which may be repeated for the occasional recurrence.

Pyogenic Granuloma

This is an inflammatory tumour caused by chronic pyogenic infection. The condition affects other parts of the skin and subcutaneous tissue but is common on the hands and fingers. It was at one time ascribed to botryomycotic infection and was called 'botryomycoma'. The theory has been proved wrong but the name is still in occasional use.

The inflammatory granulomatous tissue heaps up into a reddish, very vascular, warty or pedunculated mushroom-shaped tumour. It has a purulent discharge, but is very friable and bleeds so readily that the pus is often washed off. Cultures grow mixed pyogenic organisms, particularly *Staphylococcus aureus*. Histological examination shows the inflammatory granulations.

Treatment is by curettage and cautery followed by topical antibiotics, or by radiotherapy.

Foreign-body Granuloma

This is not uncommon in the hand. The granuloma may be frankly infected or relatively sterile. The causative foreign body may be found radiologically or only after exploration.

Mucous Cysts

These arise by mucoid degeneration in or just under the epidermis. It is likely but uncertain that trauma is the exciting agent. They occur in older individuals, particularly females, who suffer from osteoarthritis of the digital joints (Stecher and Houser, 1948). The dorsum of the distal interphalangeal joint is the most common site.

The cysts are small; they contain a colourless, mucoid fluid and have no epithelial lining. They may be multiple and bilateral (Arner, Lindholm, and Romanus, 1956).

Symptoms are slight, but the bead-like lump attracts attention. Their association with arthritis, the preponderance in women, and their situation call for differentiation from Heberden's nodes. The main point is the depth of the lesion: the mucous cyst is superficial whereas the Heberden's node begins deeper in the periarticular tissue. The subsequent ossification which occurs in the latter lesion is a further point of differentiation.

Sebaceous cysts occasionally occur on the dorsum of the hand and fingers. Their characters, the same as on other parts of the body, serve to distinguish them from mucous cysts.

Treatment is excision. Skin-grafting may be necessary when excision necessarily includes skin.

Fibroma

This occurs anywhere in the hand, but is uncommon. When it grows from a tendon-sheath or from a tendon, it disturbs the smooth gliding action of the tendon and may give rise to a 'snapping' or 'trigger' finger. Compere (1933) records a bilateral case. Otherwise, the tumours are usually symptom-free. A dubious diagnosis is settled on histological examination after the appropriate treatment, namely complete surgical removal.

Neurofibroma

This resembles a simple fibroma in its clinical presentation and the curative success of excision. Microscopy establishes the diagnosis.

Lipoma

This is also uncommon. It may involve the soft tissues, particularly in the depth of the palm, or the tendon-sheaths (Sullivan, Dahlin, and Bryan, 1956). It grows in confined spaces and tends to arborize along planes of little resistance, so that exploration often reveals a much larger and more extensive tumour than might have been anticipated on clinical grounds. Thorough exploration is required to prevent remnants being left behind; it can only be achieved by formal, adequate exposure in a bloodless field.

Angioma

Any tissue, soft or bony, of the hand and fingers may be involved. It presents as a lump and, occasionally, with discoloration of the skin. As elsewhere in the body, most of the benign lesions are hamartomata. The malignant angioma, fortunately rare, may spread rapidly and overwhelm the patient.

Glomus Tumour

Though not common, the tumour is of considerable interest and has given rise to a rich literature.

ANATOMY

Pack's description in 1939 of the detailed anatomy of a glomus body has stood the test of time. A preterminal artery, just before its break-up into capillary branches, gives off a side or shunting branch which enters a glomus, loses its elastica, and divides into several neuromuscular arterioles. The walls of these branches become thickened by an increase in smooth muscle, which remains so until an abrupt termination at the commencement of the collecting venules. Among the muscle cells are epithelioid cells or 'glomal' cells. On the venous side of the glomus these efferent glomic vessels run into a larger collecting vein. Surrounding the communicating arteriolar and venular segments in the glomus is a rich perivascular network of nerves with connexions to periarterial sympathetic nerves and also to the sensory nerves to the skin. The whole 'body' measures about 0·5–1 1 mm. in diameter.

The glomus body is situated in the stratum reticulare of the skin and probably serves the physiological function of controlled shunting of arterial blood to veins, short of the field of capillary exchange. The 'body' appears to react to stimuli for regulation of peripheral blood-flow, blood-pressure, and temperature (Lewis and Pickering, 1931).

The tumour represents hypertrophy of the glomus body.

INCIDENCE

In Boyes's (1964) series of tumours of the hands and fingers, glomus tumours account for about 1 per cent. It is roughly evenly spread in males and females, and arises at any age after childhood.

SITE

An appreciable number are subungual; most of the rest are on the hands and fingers, especially the volar pads, but any site on the surface of the body can bear the tumours.

CLINICAL PICTURE

Sharp, localized, stabbing, and severe pain is the outstanding symptom. It may be brought on by contact or by exposure to cold, or it may be spontaneous.

The pain varies from intermittent episodes to persistence for long periods; both forms may occur in one case. Although the exquisitely sharp pain remains localized, radiation of less severe pain may affect the proximal part of the limb.

Under the nail, a bluish area of about 0·5 cm. in diameter is visible and is intensely tender to light pressure. In the skin, a small nodule may or may not be palpable, but the point tenderness is highly suggestive.

The treatment, consisting of complete removal, successfully relieves pain and is not followed by recurrence.

Traumatic Neuroma

This may follow all forms of trauma to a nerve and it is not infrequently the cause of a tender amputation stump of a finger. The cut or torn nerve-fibrils grow and bunch up just distal to the proximal cut segment. There may be sufficient heaping of nerve tissue to create an appreciable tumour, or the condition is suggested by the presence of pain and tenderness at the site of the injured nerve.

The treatment of a neuroma in continuity is resection and resuture of the nerve; at the stump end of a nerve resection of the bulbous end is generally successful.

Nerve-sheath Tumours

A benign Schwannoma or neurilemmoma is an encapsulated tumour composed of modified fibrous tissue cells with a small nucleus and abundant syncytial cytoplasm. The tumours occur mainly on the volar surface of the arm and wrist. The maturity of the cells varies: the spindle cells may be plumper and have a matrix of loose reticular tissue.

The lack of differentiation of the cells is most marked in the malignant neurilemmoma. Here there is no capsule and direct spread is rapid.

The benign group tends to occur in middle age, the malignant type in younger people.

Muscle Tumours

These rare tumours of the hand may arise from smooth or striated muscle. Solitary leiomyomata have been reported (Stout, 1937) as compact, encapsulated, and subcutaneous or in the skin. The tumour and pain are the clinical directives. Excision is curative. Rhabdomyosarcoma has also been reported. It is highly malignant and the 12 cases reported by Potenza and Winslow (1961) were fatal.

Synovial Tumours

Apart from the xanthoma, or benign synovioma, discussed earlier in this chapter, there are other benign tumorous conditions arising in relation to the synovial membrane of joints and tendon-sheaths in the fingers and hands. Angiomata, fibromata, and lipomata may arise in or near a synovial lining or cavity, but they are probably only described as synovial because of the proximity of the tendon-sheath or joint; they are not derived from synovial cells and are not true synoviomata. There is doubt whether the xanthoma is, in fact, a benign synovioma. Jaffe, Lichtenstein, and Sutro (1941) argue against this view and suggest a new title to give effect to their ideas.

139

Malignant synovioma is a synovial sarcoma. It is discussed in general in Chapter 14. In the context of the present chapter, it is noteworthy that it is a rare tumour of the hand and is highly malignant.

Epidermoid Carcinoma

There are but few notable differences in the nature and behaviour of epidermoid cancers on the hands as compared with other sites on the body. It is generally the commonest cancer of man, and it is also the commonest malignant tumour affecting the hands.

The geographical and epidemiological factors, the occupational practices, and the other environmental conditions that exercise proven pathogenic influences for the cancer generally also operate as important causative agents in the hands. Exposure of sensitive skin to sunshine, ionizing radiation, certain lubricating oils like shale oil, and old scars are especially culpable as carcinogenic influences to the skin on the dorsum of the hands.

Most skin cancers occur on the head, face, and neck region; less than 1 in 10 arises in the hands (Mason, 1928). Males, being more exposed to the relevant environmental conditions, are more often affected in a ratio of about 4 : 1.

It is almost always the back of the hand that bears the lesion; occasionally the dorsum of a phalanx may be the site; more rarely it arises elsewhere. Of the epidermoid carcinomata on the hands squamous epithelioma is common; rodent cancer is rare. The cancer itself is commonly of low-grade activity, but it spreads slowly to invade deeper structures and gives late metastases, mainly to the lymphatic nodes of the axilla. It may also affect the epitrochlear node on the way. Wider spread may follow to the lungs and elsewhere.

TREATMENT

Prophylactic prevention is based on protection against the known carcinogenic agents, and on the recognition and elimination of precancerous lesions. Once cancer has begun it requires complete excision, wide of the limits of advancement of tumour cells, followed by plastic procedures for skin closure.

Carcinoma of the Nail

Most of the examples of this rare condition have followed trauma or chronic infection (Ellis, 1948). The tumour arises in the nail bed. It grows slowly, presenting in the nail fold superficially and invading the bone underneath. It gives rise to pain and is visible. The treatment is amputation of the distal phalanx.

Melanoma

It is much less common on the hands than epidermoid cancer, but there is substantial evidence that exposure to sun by very pale-skinned people is an aetiological factor (Lancaster and Nelson, 1957; Pack, Davis, and Oppenheim, 1963). Where there is more exposure to actinic rays, the peak age of presentation is in the fifth decade; in other geographical regions, the age peak rises to the sixth and seventh decades. The sexes are equally affected at all age-groups.

The status of pigmented moles as pre-melanotic lesions is very uncertain, but it has been suggested by Pack, Lenson, and Gerber (1952) and others that among the more potentially dangerous sites, moles on the palms of the hands have an increased propensity for malignant melanotic supervention.

Melanomata of the hands present the same pathological and clinical pictures and follow the same course as the tumours do in other places on the skin. There is one unique type in the fingers: the subungual lesion. A pigmented fungating and ulcerating tumour presents at the nail bed and sulcus. It often has a dark black rim around its margin. Its course is no different from other melanomata and, like others, it requires radical removal by amputation and block dissection of the axillary nodes.

BENIGN TUMOURS OF BONE

Solitary Central Chondroma or Enchondroma

About 50 per cent of these tumours occur in the hands (see Chapter 2), and it is the commonest bony tumour of the hands. The probable origin is from congenital cartilaginous rests in the bones. The main incidence occurs in the 20–30-year age-group.

CLINICAL PICTURE

A painless, fusiform swelling of one of the short tubular bones of the hand is the usual presentation. The proximal phalanges are affected most commonly, and a pathological fracture may bring the condition to first notice. The sign of 'egg-shell crackling' is found in advanced cases.

RADIOGRAPHIC PICTURE

The lesion begins at the metaphysis, then spreads to involve the diaphysis. The bone is expanded and the cortex is thinned, producing a spindle-shaped translucent swelling of the bone. The cortex may be broken through. Small foci of calcification and ossification are seen in the otherwise translucent area. Uninvolved adjacent bone is clearly demarcated from the chondroma.

Salient points in the differential diagnosis have been summarized in *Table VIII*, p. 15.

Occasionally, 'solitary enchondroma' is a misnomer, for there may be more than one short tubular bone in the hand affected. The multiplicity of bony lesions, however, does not extend to other parts of the skeleton as does the condition known as 'multiple enchondromata'.

MORBID ANATOMY AND HISTOLOGY

Islands of hyaline cartilage are set in a matrix of connective and myxomatous tissue, in which small foci of calcification and ossification are also found.

TREATMENT

The cavity of the tumour is opened, all cartilaginous and other content is curetted out. The cortex is infractured and the residual space is packed with bone chips.

Multiple Enchondromata

This is also known as 'enchondromatosis' and 'Ollier's dyschondroplasia'. The condition is generally uncommon and has no special propensity for affecting the bones of the hand. When it does, there are almost always other bones involved as well, enabling differentiation from 'solitary chondroma'.

The condition is discussed in Chapter 2.

Exostoses

These are rare on the hands. A subungual exostosis is probably initiated by trauma. Its growth is slow but it gives rise to pain at an early stage because of its pressure on the nail. Other exostoses occur in the region of the joints, following trauma in many instances.

Cysts

Simple solitary cysts occur with the same characters as elsewhere in the body (*see* Chapter 3). Exceptionally, aneurysmal bone cysts are found (Guy, Langevin, Raymond, and Martineau, 1957). Osteitis fibrosa cystica may also have one of its manifestations in a tubular bone of the hand. Chondromatous lesions may appear cystic on radiological examination, and the cytology will provide the deciding differential diagnostic criteria.

Osteoid-osteoma

This is a rare tumour in the hand, and may involve the carpal or the tubular bones. Carroll reviewed 28 cases in 1953 (Carroll, 1953b). The characters of the tumour are the same in the hand as elsewhere (*see* Chapter 3).

Benign Osteoblastoma

This is an uncommon tumour, but it has a relatively high incidence in the short tubular bones of the hands and feet, which comes second to the vertebrae in the order of site incidence. It has no special features peculiar to the hands, and the discussion in Chapter 3 is applicable here too.

Benign Fibrogenic Tumours

These are presented under several heads in Chapter 4. They seldom involve the bones of the hand and then have no locally unique characters.

MALIGNANT TUMOURS OF BONE

Chondrosarcoma

It is very rare in the bones of the hands. The tumour is the subject of Chapter 5.

Osteogenic Sarcoma

This is only an occasional tumour in the bones of the hand. In a series of 600 cases reported by Dahlin and Coventry (1967), there were 3 cases, i.e., 0·5 per cent, in the hands. It may be a primary lesion or secondary to a benign tumour. Carroll's paper in 1957 includes 2 personal and 8 recorded cases. He agrees with other opinions that the prognosis in the hand is more favourable than it is elsewhere.

The subject is featured in Chapter 6.

Fibrosarcoma

This may occur in bony or soft tissues; in the latter site it may distort and invade adjacent bone.

Trauma has been inculpated but its place is subject to question.

The tumour is very rare in the hands and diagnosis depends upon histological examination.

Giant-cell Tumour

The tumour is discussed in Chapter 9; its characters, when it occasionally occurs in the hand, are no different from those already described. Ionizing radiation therapy is disadvantageous and is contra-indicated for this as it is for most conditions of the hand.

Ewing's Sarcoma

The hand is an exceptional site for this rather uncommon tumour. In the hand, it follows the pattern exhibited elsewhere (*see* Chapter 10).

Kaposi's Sarcoma

As has been indicated in the discussion of Kaposi's sarcoma in Chapter 12, the condition frequently involves bone and may, in fact, take origin in bone. Of the bones affected, those of the hands and feet are the most common and the earliest to suffer. The initial peripheral site of the lesions in bone corresponds to the distribution in the skin.

The peculiarities of geographical distribution and other aspects of aetiology, pathology, and the clinical features of bone involvement are reviewed in Chapter 12. It remains to add a note on the skin manifestations, which commonly appear on the hands. These evidences, together with the bony lesions, often clinch the diagnosis.

In white patients, the first skin signs are dark blue to violaceous macules, often with a brown tint. Infiltrated plaques replace the macules; then nodules appear, measuring 0·5-3 cm. in diameter. Some lesions may undergo healing; others may coalesce and ulcerate. Most commonly, the feet show the first skin lesions; quite often, it is the hands that are the earliest sites; and sometimes both hands and feet are affected together. The manifestations subsequently appear at progressively more proximal levels, each crop starting with the early discoloured macule, so producing a series of lesions exhibiting different stages of development.

Metastatic Carcinoma

Such metastases are very exceptional. Most of those reported in the literature have come from primary bronchogenic cancers. The clinical suggestion of an inflammatory condition of a phalanx may acquire further, though false, suppor from the radiological picture of an osteolytic focus. An erroneous diagnosis, and consequently unsatisfactory treatment, is the more likely because the rarity of metastatic cancer in these bones blunts the observer's awareness of its existence.

REFERENCES

ARNER, O., LINDHOLM, A., and ROMANUS, R. (1956), 'Mucous Cysts of the Fingers; 26 Cases', *Acta chir. scand.*, **111**, 314.

BOYES, J. H. (1964), *Bunnell's Surgery of the Hand*, 4th ed. Philadelphia: Lippincott.

CARP, L., and STOUT, A. P. (1928), 'Study of Ganglion with Especial Reference to Treatment', *Surgery Gynec. Obstet.*, **47**, 460.

CARROLL, R. E. (1953a), 'Epidermoid (Epithelial) Cyst of the Hand Skeleton', *Am. J. Surg.*, **85**, 327.

— — (1953b), 'Osteoid Osteoma in the Hand', *J. Bone Jt Surg.*, **35A**, 888.

— — (1957), 'Osteogenic Sarcoma in the Hand', *Ibid.*, **39A**, 325.

COMPERE, E. L. (1933), 'Bilateral Snapping Thumbs', *Ann. Surg.*, **97**, 773.

DAHLIN, D. C., and COVENTRY, M. B. (1967), 'Osteogenic Sarcoma', *J. Bone Jt Surg.*, **49A**, 101.

ELLIS, V. H. (1948), 'Squamous-cell Carcinoma of the Nail Bed', *Ibid.*, **30B**, 656.

GUY, R., LANGEVIN, R., RAYMOND, O., and MARTINEAU, G. (1957), 'Phalangeal Aneurysmal Bone Cyst', *Un. méd. Can.*, **86**, 866.

JAFFE, H. L., LICHTENSTEIN, L., and SUTRO, C. J. (1941), 'Pigmented Villonodular Synovitis, Bursitis, and Tenosynovitis', *Archs Path.*, **31**, 731.

KING, E. S. J. (1933), 'Post-traumatic Epidermoid Cysts of Hands and Fingers', *Br. J. Surg.*, **21**, 29.

LANCASTER, H. O., and NELSON, J. (1957), 'Sunlight as a Cause of Melanoma: A Clinical Survey', *Aust. med. J.*, **1**, 452.

LEWIS, T., and PICKERING, G. W. (1931), 'Vasodilatation in the Limbs in Response to warming the Body with Evidence for Sympathetic Vasodilator Nerves in Man', *Heart*, **16**, 33.

MASON, M. L. (1928), 'Carcinoma of the Hand', *Archs Surg., Chicago*, **18**, 2107.

PACK, G. T. (1939), *Tumors of the Hands and Feet*. St. Louis: Mosby.

— — DAVIS, J., and OPPENHEIM, A. (1963), 'Relation of Race and Complexion to Incidence of Moles and Melanoma', *Ann. N.Y. Acad. Sci.*, **100**, 719.

— — LENSON, N., and GERBER, D. M. (1952), 'Regional Distribution of Moles and Melanomas', *Archs Surg., Chicago*, **65**, 862.

PHALEN, G. S., McCORMACK, L. J., and GAZALE, W. J. (1959), 'Giant-cell Tumour of the Tendon Sheath (Benign Synovioma) in the Hand. Evaluation of 56 Cases', *Clin. Orthop.*, **15**, 140.

POTENZA, A., and WINSLOW, D. (1961), 'Rhabdomyosarcoma of the Hand', *J. Bone Jt Surg.*, **43A**, 700.

STECHER, R. M., and HOUSER, H. (1948), 'Heberden's Nodes', *Am. J. Roent.*, **59**, 326.

STOUT, A. P. (1937), 'Solitary Cutaneous and Subcutaneous Leiomyoma', *Am. J. Cancer*, **29**, 435.

SULLIVAN, C. R., DAHLIN, D. C., and BRYAN, R. S. (1956), 'Lipoma of the Tendon Sheath', *J. Bone Jt Surg.*, **38A**, 1275.

INDEX

PAGE

'ACANTHOMATOUS ameloblastoma' .. 129
'Aclasis, diaphysial' 22
Adamantinoma 126, 128
— of tibia 102
Adeno-ameloblastoma 130
Adrenalectomy in treatment of breast
   cancer 110
Age incidence of tumours 5
Albright's disease 37
Alkaline phosphatase in diagnosis of
   tumour 7
— — raised 55
Ameloblastic fibroma 131
— haemangioma 131
— odontoma 131
Ameloblastoma 126, 128
Anaemia 66, 83, 90
Androgen treatment of breast cancer .. 109
Aneurysmal bone cyst .. (Fig. 5), 31, 33, 80
— — — of jaw 127
— — — vertebrae 121
Angioblastoma 102
Angioma of hand 138
Angiosarcoma 100
Anorexia 90
Apical cysts 124
Arthritis 22, 66

BENCE-JONES protein 91
Biopsy 7–8
Bone abscess, cortical, differential diagnosis of (Table XVII) 44
— — differential diagnosis of (Table XIII) 28
— aneurysm, malignant 57
— changes due to metastases 108
— cyst, aneurysmal .. (Fig. 5) 31, 33, 80
— — — of jaw 127
— — — vertebrae 121
— — solitary .. .. (Fig. 5) 31, 80
— — — of jaw 127
— fibrosarcoma of, differential diagnosis
   of .. .. .. (Table XXII) 58
— formation, new 7
— haemangioma of 35
— irradiated, sarcoma in 65
— Kaposi's sarcoma of 100, 143
— lesions associated with malignant neoplasms of haemopoietic tissues
   (Fig. 14; Tables XXXIII–XXXV) 89
— — secondary, in reticulum-cell sarcoma 96
— malignant vascular tumours of .. 99

PAGE

Bone metastases, site of .. (Fig. 15) 107
— metastatic carcinoma of
   (Fig. 15; Table XXXVI) 106
— neural tumours of 36
— sarcoma, dial painter's .. (Fig. 10) 66
— — Registry of .. .. .. (Table I) 1
— tumours, benign fibrogenic 37
— — — of hand 141
— — differential diagnosis of primary
   and metastatic (Table XXXVI) 108
— — incidence of .. (Table V) 4–5
— — malignant, of hand 142
Bone-marrow tumours 97–8
Botryomycoma 136
Breast cancers metastasizing to bone 106, 109
Burkitt's tumour 128, 134

CALVARIUM, haemangioma of 36
Cancer, ossophile, metastasizing to bone 106
Carcinoma, epidermoid, of hand .. 140
— metastatic anaplastic 96
— — in bone (Fig. 15; Table XXXVI) 106
— — differential diagnosis of
   (Tables XXIV, XXV) 59, 92, 93
— — of hand 143
— — vertebral column 118
— squamous-cell 68
Cartilage lesions, calcified, and fibrosarcoma 73
— neoplasm involving bone 75
Cementifying fibroma 138
Cementoma 131
Chloroma 89, 90
Chondroblastoma, benign
   (Fig. 1; Tables VI, VII) 10–12
— — differential diagnosis of
   (Tables VI, VII) 12
Chondroma 1
— chondrosarcoma secondary to .. 52
— periosteal, differential diagnosis of
   (Table X) 44
— solitary central .. .. (Fig. 2) 12
— — — of hand 141
— of vertebra 121
Chondromatosis, synovial 112
Chondromyxoid fibroma 40, 48, 72
Chondrosarcoma 1, 7, 39
— age incidence of 5
— central 7
— — differential diagnosis of
   (Tables VII, XXIII) 12, 58
— of hand 142

PAGE

Chondrosarcoma, primary central   (*Fig.* 7) 46
— — peripheral ..   (*Tables XIX, XX*) 49
— secondary to chondroma   52
— — differential diagnosis of   (*Table XX*) 50
— — to osteochondroma   (*Table XX*) 50
— of vertebrae   120
Chordoma   103
— of vertebrae   120
Classification of tumours   (*Tables I–III*) 1–4
Codman's triangle 55, 108
Constipation   104
Cortical expansion   108
Cysts, epidermoid inclusion   136
— follicular   125
— of hand   142
— jaw, surgical treatment of   127
— mucous, of hand   137
— non-odontogenic tumorous   127
— odontogenic, benign   124
— radicular   124
— vestigial epithelial   126

DENTAL cysts   124
Dentigerous cyst   125
Dentinoma   130
Desmoplastic fibroma   45
Dial painter's bone sarcoma   ..   (*Fig.* 10) 66
'Diaphysial aclasis'   22
Diarrhoea   104
Dyschondroplasia, Ollier's (*see* Enchon-
   droma, multiple)
Dysplasia   3
— fibrous (*see* Fibrous Dysplasia)

'EGG-SHELL crackling' 14, 77
Enchondroma 1, 3, 6, 12, 48
— differential diagnosis of   (*Table IX*) 12, 48
— multiple   15
— — differential diagnosis of   (*Table XI*) 24
— — of hand   142
— solitary ..   ..   (*Fig.* 2) 12
Enchondromatosis (*see* Enchondroma,
   multiple)
Eosinophilic granuloma, differential diagnosis of   ..   (*Table XXIX*) 84, 86
Ependymoma   122
Epidermoid carcinoma of hand   140
— inclusion cysts   136
Epithelial cyst   125
— — vestigial   126
Ewing's sarcoma
   (*Fig.* 13; *Tables XXVIII–XXXII*) 58, 82, 95
— — differential diagnosis of   (*Table XXX*) 84
— — of hand   143
— — jaw   133
— — vertebrae   121
Exostosis of hand   142

PAGE

Exostosis, hereditary 3, 6
— of jaw   131
— osteocartilaginous   ..   ..   (*Fig.* 3) 19
Extra-skeletal osteogenic sarcoma   ..   68

FIBROCYSTIC disease (*see* Fibrous Dysplasia)
Fibrogenic tumours, benign, of bone   ..   37
— — — hand   142
Fibrolipoma   116
Fibroma, ameloblastic   131
— cementifying   131
— chondromyxoid 40, 48, 72
— desmoplastic 45, 72
— of hand   137
— jaws   130
— non-ossifying, differential diagnosis of
   (*Table XVIII*) 45, 80
— non-osteogenic 41, 72
— osteogenic   29
Fibromyxolipoma   116
Fibrosarcoma   ..   (*Fig.* 11) 45, 68, 70, 116
— of bone, differential diagnosis of
   (*Table XXII*) 58
— hand   143
— parosteal   73
— periosteal (*see* Fibrosarcoma, parosteal)
— primary   ..   ..   (*Table XXII*) 72
— secondary   73
— of vertebrae   121
Fibrous cortical defect   ..   ..   (*Fig.* 6) 41
— — — differential diagnosis of
   (*Tables X, XVII*) 28
— dysplasia 37, 72
— — of jaw   132
— — monostotic   32
— — — differential diagnosis of
   (*Table XXI*) 58
— — sarcoma in   68
— — and solitary bone cyst   32
— — of vertebrae   121
Follicular cysts   125
— — ameloblastoma associated with   ..   128
Foreign-body granuloma   137

GANGLION   116
— of hand   135
Geschickter's classification of tumours   ..   2
Giant-cell reparative granuloma of jaw   132
— tumour (*Fig.* 12; *Table XXVII*) 6, 7, 76, 113
— — differential diagnosis of
   (*Tables VI, IX, XVI, XXVII*) 35
— — of hand   143
— — jaw   132
— — sarcoma in   68
— — of tendon-sheath   116
— — — differential diagnosis of (*Table X*) 19
— — of vertebrae   121

PAGE

Globomaxillary cyst 126
Glomus tumour of hand 138
Granuloma, dental 124
— eosinophilic, differential diagnosis of
(*Table XXIX*) 32, 84, 86
— foreign-body, of hand 137
— healing, differential diagnosis of
(*Table XXVII*) 79
— pyogenic, of hand 136

HAEMANGIOMA 17
— ameloblastic 131
— associated with multiple enchondromata 16
— of bone 35
— synovial 112
— of vertebrae 121
Haemangiosarcoma 99
Haemopoietic tissues, malignant neoplasms of, associated with bone
lesions
(*Fig.* 14; *Tables XXXIII–XXXV*) 89
Hand, benign bone tumours of 141
— malignant bone tumours of 142
— metastatic carcinoma of 143
— tumours of 135
Heberden's nodes 137
Hodgkin's disease 89, 96
— — and Kaposi's sarcoma 101
Hypercalcaemia 90
Hyperparathyroidism 7, 39
— differential diagnosis of
(*Tables XXXIV, XXVII*) 79, 92
— and solitary bone cyst 32
Hypertension 66
Hyperthyroidism 38
Hypophysectomy in treatment of breast
cancer 110

INCLUSION cysts, epidermoid 136
Inflammatory conditions 60
Irradiated bone, sarcoma in 65

JAFFE's classification of tumours (*Table II*) 1–2
Jaw cysts, surgical treatment of 127
— exostosis of 131
— malignant tumours of 132
— metastatic tumours of 134
— odontogenic tumours of 128
— tumours of 123
Juxtacortical sarcoma 7

KAPOSI's sarcoma of bone 100, 101, 143
Kidney cancer metastasizing to bone 106, 111

LESIONS, solitary, in long bones (*Table IX*) 16
— — short-long bones .. (*Table VIII*) 15

PAGE

Leukaemia and Kaposi's sarcoma .. 101
— lymphocytic 97
— myelocytic 89
— myelogenous 97–8
Lipoma 116
— of hand 137
Liposarcoma involving bone 75
Long bones, solitary lesions in (*Table IX*) 16
Lung cancer metastasizing to bone 106, 111
Lymphoma 82
— of bone, malignant .. (*Fig.* 14) 89, 94
— and Kaposi's sarcoma 101
— of vertebrae 121
Lymphoreticular neoplasia 89
Lymphosarcoma 89, 97
— and Kaposi's sarcoma 101

MAFFUCCI's syndrome 16
Malformation 3
Maxilla, median fissural cysts of .. 126
Medullary osteoma, differential diagnosis
of .. .. .. (*Table XII*) 27
Melano-ameloblastoma 130
Melanoma of hand 140
Mental aberration 90
Metastases to bone, site of (*Fig.* 15) 107
Metastatic carcinoma of hand 143
— tumours of jaw 134
Mucous cysts of hand 137
Multilocular cyst 125
Muscle neoplasm involving bone .. 75
— tumours in hand 139
— wasting 10
Muscular weakness 90
Mycosis fungoides and Kaposi's sarcoma 101
Myeloma 7
— of jaw 133
— multiple (*Tables XXXIV, XXXV*) 90
— plasma-cell 90
— of vertebrae 120
Myelomatosis (*Tables XXXIV, XXXV*) 90
Myositis ossificans, differential diagnosis of
(*Table XXVI*) 64
Myxoma 130

NAIL, carcinoma of 140
Nasopalatine cysts 127
Nausea 90
Neoplasia 3
Neoplasms of haemopoietic tissues, malig-
nant, bone lesions associated with
(*Fig.* 14; *Tables XXXIII–XXXV*) 89
— in osteomyelitis 68
Nerve-sheath tumours 139
Neural tumours of bone 36
Neurilemmoma 131, 139
— of vertebrae 121

PAGE

Neuroblastoma metastasizing to bone .. 110
— metastatic, differential diagnosis of
(*Table XXXII*) 85, 87
Neurofibroma of hand 137
Neurofibromatosis 36
Neuroma, traumatic 139

ODONTOGENIC apparatus, tumours of .. 123
— cyst 125
— — benign 124
— tumours of jaw 128
Odontoma 131
— epithelial 128
— soft 128
Oestrogen treatment of breast cancer .. 110
Oliguria 90
Ollier's dyschondroplasia (*see* Enchondroma, multiple)
Oophorectomy in treatment of breast
cancer 110
Ossophile cancers metastasizing to bone.. 106
Osteitis deformans, Paget's 3, 7
— fibrosa (*see* Fibrous Dysplasia)
— radiation, and fibrosarcoma 73
Osteoblastic metastases 108
Osteoblastoma 6
— benign .. .. .. (*Fig.* 4) 27, 29
— — of hand 142
— — vertebrae 121
Osteocartilaginous exostosis (*Fig.* 3) 6, 19, 21
Osteochondroma 64
— chondrosarcoma secondary to (*Table XX*) 50
— multiple, differential diagnosis of
(*Table XIX*) 49
— solitary .. .. .. (*Fig.* 3) 6, 19, 21
Osteochondromatosis 112
— multiple, differential diagnosis of
(*Table XI*) 21
Osteoclastoma (*see* Giant-cell Tumour) .. 76
Osteogenic fibroma 29
— sarcoma
(*Fig.* 8; *Tables XXI–XXIV*) 1, 7, 39, 46, 53
— — age incidence of 5
— — differential diagnosis of
(*Tables XIV, XXI–XXV, XXXI*) 28, 48, 62,
85, 87
— — extra-skeletal 68
— — of hand 142
— — juxtacortical
(*Fig.* 9; *Tables XXV, XXVI*) 62
— — osteolytic .. .. (*Table XXII*) 72
— — parosteal 62
— — telangiectatic 34
— — of vertebrae 121
Osteoid-osteoma (*Fig.* 4; *Tables XII–XV*) 26
— differential diagnosis of
(*Tables XII–XV, XVII*) 30, 44, 58

PAGE

Osteoid-osteoma, giant 29
— of hand 142
— jaw 132
— vertebrae 121
Osteolytic activity of tumours 7
— metastases 108
— osteogenic sarcoma .. (*Table XXII*) 72
Osteoma, medullary, differential diagnosis
of .. .. .. (*Table XII*) 27
— parosteal 62
Osteomyelitis 6, 83
— chronic 35
— differential diagnosis of
(*Tables XIII, XXVIII*) 28, 84, 85
— neoplasm in 68

PAGET's disease and fibrosarcoma .. 73
— — sarcoma in .. .. (*Fig.* 10) 67
— osteitis deformans 3, 7
Pain in diagnosis of tumour 6
Paraplegia 36
Periodontal cysts 124, 125
Pigmented villonodular synovitis
(*Table XXXVII*) 113, 116, 136
Plasma-cell myeloma 90
Plasmocytoma 92
Primordial cyst 125
Prostate cancer metastazing to bone 106, 110
Puberty, precocious 38
Pyogenic granuloma 136

RADIATION osteitis and fibrosarcoma .. 73
Radicular cysts 124
Radioactive drugs, internal 66
Radiograph, shadow densities on .. 7
— 'soap-bubble' 7
Radiographic evidence of tumour .. 7–8
Registry of Bone Sarcoma .. (*Table I*) 1
Rest-pain 6
Reticular system malignancy, bone lesions
associated with
(*Fig.* 14; *Tables XXXIII–XXXV*) 89
Reticulum-cell sarcoma (*Fig.* 14) 59, 92, 89, 94
— — differential diagnosis of
(*Table XXX*) 85, 86
— — secondary bone lesions in .. 96
Rhabdomyosarcoma 139
Rheumatic fever 97

SARCOMA (*see also specific sarcomata*)
— Bone, Registry of .. .. (*Table I*) 1
— in irradiated bone 65
— of jaw .. .. (*Table XXXVIII*) 133
— in Paget's disease .. .. (*Fig.* 10) 67
— site of predilection of 6
Schwannoma 36, 139
Scoliosis 36

PAGE

Sequestration, non-odontogenic 126
Serum calcium level in diagnosis of
    tumour 7
— protein, derangement of 90
Sexual precocity 38
Short-long bones, solitary lesions in
                (*Table VIII*) 15
Site of predilection of tumours 6
Soft-tissue sarcoma, extension from .. 75
Solitary bone cyst of jaw 127
Squamous-cell carcinoma 68
Still's disease 97
Synovial chondromatosis 112
— haemangioma 112
— sarcoma .. (*Table XXXVII*) 114
— tumours of hand 139
Synovioma, benign 113
— malignant .. (*Table XXXVII*) 114
Synovium neoplasm involving bone .. 75
— tumours of .. (*Table XXXVII*) 112
Synovitis 135
— pigmented villonodular
      (*Table XXXVII*) 113, 116, 136
Syphilis 6, 7

Telangiectatic osteogenic sarcoma .. 34
Tendon-sheath, giant-cell tumour of
            (*Table X*) 44, 116
— — — differential diagnosis of (*Table X*) 19
— haemangioma 113
Tenosynovitis 135
Thyroid cancer metastasizing to bone 106, 110
Tibia, adamantinoma of 102
Torus 131
Traumatic conditions 60

PAGE

Tumours (*see also individual tumours*)
— benign non-odontogenic 131
— chondrogenic, differential diagnosis of
          (*Tables VI–XI*) 10
— classification of .. (*Tables I–III*) 1–4
— clinical features of 5–7
— diagnosis of 5–9
— history of, as aid to diagnosis .. 6
— incidence of .. .. (*Tables IV, V*) 4–5
— malignant, of vertebrae 34
— osteogenic benign 26
— primary and secondary 1
— progress of, as aid to diagnosis .. 5
— radiographic evidence of 7–8
— site of 6
— size of, as aid to diagnosis 7
— soft-tissue, of hand 135
— of synovium .. (*Table XXXVII*) 112
Typhoid fever 6

Urinary disturbances 104

Vascular tumours of bone, malig-
    nant 99
Vertebrae, haemangioma of 35
— malignant tumours of 34
Vertebral column, tumours of 118
— metastases, mechanisms of .. 118–19
Vessel neoplasm involving bone 75
Villonodular synovitis, pigmented
      (*Table XXXVII*) 113, 116, 136

White-cell count in diagnosis of tumour 7

Xanthoma 113, 136